Combining Medication and Psychosocial
Treatments for Addictions

Combining Medication and Psychosocial Treatments for Addictions

The BRENDA Approach

Joseph R. Volpicelli
Helen M. Pettinati
A. Thomas McLellan
Charles P. O'Brien

Foreword by William R. Miller

The Guilford Press
New York   London

© 2001 The Guilford Press
A Division of Guilford Publications, Inc.
72 Spring Street, New York, NY 10012
www.guilford.com

Printed in the United States of America

This book is printed on acid-free paper.

Last digit is print number: 9   8   7   6   5   4   3   2   1

Library of Congress Cataloging-in-Publication Data

Combining medication and psychosocial treatments for addictions :
the BRENDA approach / Joseph R. Volpicelli . . . [et al.]
    p.   cm.
   Includes bibliographical references and index.
   ISBN 1-57230-618-1
   1. Drug abuse—Chemotherapy. 2. Narcotic addicts—Counseling of.
  3. Combined modality therapy. I. Volpicelli, Joseph.
   [DNLM: 1. Substance-Related Disorders—therapy. 2. Combined
Modality Therapy. 3. Drug Therapy—methods. 4. Patient Compliance.
5. Psychotherapy—methods. WM270
C7313   2001]
RC564 .C645 2001
616.86′06—dc21   00-069163

About the Authors

Joseph R. Volpicelli, MD, PhD, is Associate Professor of Psychiatry and Psychology at the University of Pennsylvania and Senior Scientist at the University of Pennsylvania/Veterans Administration (Penn/VA) Center for Studies of Addiction. He has authored over 100 publications on studies of the behavioral and biochemical aspects of addictions and has recently published the book *Recovery Options: The Complete Guide*. He developed the use of naltrexone for the treatment of alcoholism and has received several clinical, teaching, and research awards, including the Joel Elks International Award in Neuropsychopharmacology for his research into the study of the pharmacology of addictions.

Helen M. Pettinati, PhD, is a Research Associate Professor of Psychiatry in the University of Pennsylvania School of Medicine and the Director of the Treatment Research Division at the University of Pennsylvania/ Veterans Administration (Penn/VA) Center for Studies of Addiction. She has conducted clinical research and published extensively on substance abuse/dependence, depression, psychopharmacology, treatment non-compliance, and measuring outcome. Her current research targets new treatments for substance-dependent patients with comorbid psychiatric disorders, part of which includes examining medication combinations, and also combining medications with various kinds of psychosocial interventions.

A. Thomas McLellan, PhD, is a psychologist at the Philadelphia Veterans Affairs Medical Center, Professor of Psychiatry at the University of Pennsylvania, and the Director of the Treatment Research Institute in Philadelphia. He has published more than 300 articles and chapters in addiction research. Dr. McLellan and his colleagues have been developing and evaluating treatments for alcohol and drug dependence as well as evaluation instruments such as the Addiction Severity Index (ASI) and the Treatment Services Review (TSR). They are currently pursuing questions such as "What are the active and inactive ingredients of treatment?" and "What is the appropriate duration and content of treatment for various types of patients?"

Charles P. O'Brien, MD, PhD, is Chief of Psychiatry at the Philadelphia Veterans Affairs Medical Center, Professor and Vice-Chairman of Psychiatry at the University of Pennsylvania, and Director of the University of Pennsylvania/Veterans Administration (Penn/VA) Center for Studies of Addiction. Certified in neurology, psychiatry, and addiction psychiatry, his research interests include the psychopharmacology of addiction and the development of new behavioral and pharmacological treatments for addiction, including alcoholism, using controlled clinical trials. He has authored more than 400 publications in the area of addictive disorders and biological psychiatry. Dr. O'Brien's addiction research has been recognized by numerous awards, an honorary doctorate from the University of Bordeaux, and election to the Institute of Medicine of the National Academy of Sciences.

Acknowledgments

We would like to thank the staff of the University of Pennsylvania's Treatment Research Center who helped cultivate the BRENDA approach, especially the Center's excellent clinicians—namely, Louise Epperson, Gail Kaempf, Moira Molloy, and Janice Biddle—for providing valuable feedback throughout BRENDA's development. We also owe a large intellectual debt to other scientists outside our Center who helped shape the ideas that form the basis of this book, especially William Miller and his work on motivational enhancement for the treatment of addictions, and Ron Ulm, a colleague who for over two decades supported and provided valuable input into understanding addictions as a biopsychosocial disorder. We also thank the many people who helped in the writing of this manual, especially Heather Wallace, Maia Szalavitz, and the invaluable comments of our senior editor Barbara Watkins at The Guilford Press. We also acknowledge the National Institute on Alcohol Abuse and Alcoholism and the National Institute on Drug Abuse for consistently funding our program of research. Finally, we acknowledge the support of our friends and families who have encouraged us at each step.

Preface

The idea for writing this book was first conceived 5 years ago. It was late summer and a tumultuous thunderstorm had just uprooted a tree and left several large branches lying on the ground. What caught my attention was the lack of damage to the willow trees. During the storm, the trees with stiff rigid branches broke while the branches of willow trees were flexible enough to accommodate the wind. I thought of my work with several patients who failed in their previous attempts to recover from their addictions. Their comments of their previous treatment experiences reminded me of the rigid trees unable to accommodate to the storm. I decided to take a different approach. Like the willow tree, I applied a less rigid approach and attempted to accommodate my therapy to the patients' needs. Borrowing from ideas on the psychology of improving one's motivation to change, from the understanding that behavioral changes occur in various stages, and from the biopsychosocial approach to understanding addictions that guides the teaching at the University of Pennsylvania, the BRENDA approach was born.

My colleagues and I found that by listening to patients, we could gather data on how alcohol and drug use led to biopsychosocial complications across various aspects of the patients' lives. In a nonconfrontational manner, we simply reported back the results of the evaluation and related how alcohol drinking or drug use was complicating their lives. Often this was enough to motivate patients to take steps to address their problems. But some patients remained ambivalent. Treating patients with respect and empathy, we attempted to understand the disorder from the patients' perspective. Only after understanding the patients' needs did we offer direct advice and recommendations on how to best meet their needs. For some people, the advice was well received and people adhered to the treatment recommendations. Often, however, patients ignored or did not follow through with treatment recommendations. Rather than blame the patients, we tried to understand why. Usually this discussion led to a better understanding of the patients' needs and improved treatment recommendations that were more likely to be utilized.

Addiction counselors, psychologists, nurse practitioners, and other health care professionals have found this approach easy to learn and helpful in retaining patients in treatment and improving medication adherence. The motivation to write this book was to introduce this approach to other health care professionals who wish to treat addictions using a flexible biopsychosocial approach that easily accommodates the use of medications.

JOSEPH R. VOLPICELLI

Foreword

The need for a structured treatment like BRENDA is evident. Both scientific knowledge and the treatment of addictions have changed markedly in recent years. Addictive behaviors have begun to lose their former mystique as a strange disease requiring intensive treatment that can be provided only by specialists with unique expertise. Instead, it has become clearer that these are behaviors, and as such respond to the same psychological principles of motivation, learning, and cognition that have been applied successfully in the treatment of so many other problems. An increasingly complex biopsychosocial understanding of addictions has led to the demise of many prior black-and-white conceptions. The unique-disease notion that either "you have it or you don't" has given way to approaches that address a continuum of severity of use, problems, and dependence. The all-or-none concept of "relapse" is being replaced by an understanding that recovery is usually characterized by successive steps in the right direction. Instead of insisting on immediate and lifelong abstinence as the only successful outcome, there is a recognition that much can be done to reduce harm before total abstinence is achieved. Whereas the use of medications in treatment was once shunned, it is now recognized that pharmacotherapy can contribute significantly to the achievement and stability of sobriety.

Most professionals reject a simplistic notion of pharmacotherapy for addictions, that "all you have to do is prescribe." Medications are seen as a supplement to, not a replacement for, other treatment. It is also the case that without other support, compliance with medication tends to be poor.

That's where BRENDA has much to teach us. How can health professionals combine pharmacotherapy with effective counseling approaches? What can be done to increase adherence to a prescribed medication? What happens if the person is not abstaining? What about the other needs that invariably arise during treatment? Where is the optimal balance between support and directiveness? These are important practical questions that arise as pharmacotherapies and psychosocial approaches are combined in the treatment and management of addictions.

BRENDA brings together some of the important scientific evidence and clinical innovations of the late 20th century. It incorporates the transtheoretical model of change, the empathic yet directive style of motivational interviewing, feedback of evaluation results to the patient, and practical principles of case management. It is adaptable to many forms of drug abuse, and can be used both with currently available pharmacotherapies and with new medications as they emerge. As addictive behaviors are increasingly addressed within health care and social service settings, this is the way treatment is likely to be done in the 21st century. In this book, practical case examples are provided to show how BRENDA speaks to people in the clinic, and session outlines are offered to illustrate the course of treatment.

There are some caveats, of course. BRENDA is not in itself a comprehensive treatment approach, but rather a framework for management of addictions. It is, in a way, a good beginning for recovery, whether or not further treatment is obtained. It is compatible with a variety of other treatment approaches, and is designed to get people started on the right course. At present the authors do not have controlled trial evidence for the efficacy of this approach. To date it has been used successfully as a platform upon which to test the efficacy of pharmacotherapies, and the specific benefits of BRENDA itself now need to be demonstrated. Based on what we do know about what works in managing addictions, however, it is a sensible approach. The publication of this clinician manual will now allow for specific testing and replication.

I am both excited and concerned about the obvious trend, under managed care, toward managing substance use disorders within health care settings. In many ways it is a natural and sensible direction. People with alcohol and other drug problems are more likely to turn up in the health care system than in specialist treatment programs. Health care professionals will be treating people with addictions, whether we know it (and know how) or not. Substance use disorders contribute to, complicate, even cause many of the problems that prompt them to seek health care. There is often substantial reluctance, at least at first, to accept formal treatment. There is strong evidence that brief interventions, of a magnitude compatible with health care delivery, are substantially more effective than not addressing these problems at all. In all these ways, it seems like a good idea.

So what, then, are my concerns? They are several. Most of us who deliver health care are already quite busy with, if not overwhelmed by, the demands of practice in the era of managed care. Adding one more complicated problem area and protocol to an already overstretched practice can seem unmanageable. The effective treatment of substance use disorders is also rather different from the treatment of acute illnesses. An authoritative, directive approach often bombs. I fear that the dispensing of medications for addictions could be thought of much as the prescription of antibiotics for infections. There are common features, of course, such as problems with medication adherence, but addictions center not on an invasive organism, but on a pervasive behavior. A busy schedule and a mind-set to treating acute illnesses can easily combine to produce a "Just do it!" approach that frustrates both patient and practitioner, and becomes a self-perpetuating cycle.

Quite different from that approach is BRENDA's patient, structured, empathic style of counseling. The busy clinician sometimes protests that "I don't have time for that!" In truth, we don't have time not to listen to our patients. A little bit of good, empathic listening goes a long way, and is more likely to motivate change than any course of finger-wagging advice. That's what I hope doesn't get lost in this transition, and in the practice of health care more generally.

WILLIAM R. MILLER, PHD
Distinguished Professor of Psychology
and Psychiatry
The University of New Mexico

Contents

PART I

The BRENDA Approach
and How to Use It

CHAPTER 1

The Biopsychosocial Understanding of Addiction

This manual describes a simple, six-stage framework for integrating the use of medications in the treatment of people with alcohol and drug addiction. This approach, based on a biopsychosocial model of addictions, is unique in its integrated use of both pharmacotherapy and individualized psychosocial support and services. The manual incorporates the motivation-enhancing techniques originally suggested by Miller and associates (Miller, 1998) and focuses on the role of the collaborative relationship between the treatment provider and patient to enhance treatment adherence and improve treatment outcomes. In addition, it incorporates specific information on medications recently developed for treating addictions, with a special focus on naltrexone in the treatment of alcohol dependence. The program outlined here is relatively simple to learn and has been used clinically for over 5 years in our Treatment Research Center by nurse practitioners with no specialized addiction treatment training. Successful treatment outcomes have been obtained in over 80% of the alcohol-dependent referrals to our program using the six stages of the framework, together with referrals and prescriptions for coexisting medical or psychiatric problems (Kaempf, O'Donnell, et al., 1999; Pettinati, Volpicelli, et al., 2000). We

3

call the approach described in this manual BRENDA, an acronym for the six stages of this care management framework:

1. **B**iopsychosocial evaluation
2. **R**eport to the patient on assessment
3. **E**mpathetic understanding of the patient's situation
4. **N**eeds collaboratively identified by the patient and treatment provider
5. **D**irect advice to patient on how to meet those needs
6. **A**ssess reaction of the patient to advice and adjust as necessary for best care

Each of these stages is discussed in detail later in this book. This model emphasizes a collaborative, case-management approach to treatment. Based on an initial biopsychosocial assessment, the BRENDA provider selects and arranges those treatment options most suited to the individual patient. In many but not all cases, the BRENDA manager may directly provide a treatment while also coordinating services by other providers as needed. Through this approach, work by addiction counselors, psychologists, family therapists, physicians, nurses, and/or social workers can be coordinated into an individualized treatment program specific to the individual needs of the person presenting for treatment. If your training is in addiction counseling, and you do not have medical training, this manual describes the advantages of adding medications to improve treatment outcomes and how your treatment can be integrated with pharmacotherapy. For medically trained practitioners, this manual describes when and how you may need to refer to mental health care providers to address the emotional and behavioral problems that complicate the addiction.

Persons with drug and alcohol problems can initially present to a variety of health care providers. Physicians, nurse practitioners, psychologists, counselors, and social workers each have key roles to play in identifying and managing treatment of alcohol and drug addiction. You need not be an addiction specialist to manage care within the BRENDA approach but it is crucial that you have a basic understanding of substance addiction and of the special needs of these individuals. Specifically, you must be able to

- Accurately understand the difference between recreational use of a drug and addiction
- Conduct a thorough biopsychosocial evaluation
- Monitor progress in treatment
- Have an empathetic, nonjudgmental approach toward individuals who are presenting for treatment
- Motivate the patient and facilitate cooperation between treatment providers and patients.

This manual provides a method for integrating various "tools" of treatment. We do not expect each care provider to be an expert; however, after mastering the concepts in this manual, you should be able to coordinate a team of providers to optimize treatment outcomes.

A REVIEW OF TRADITIONAL ADDICTION TREATMENTS

The history of treatment for substance addiction has been marked by a clash of ideas about the nature of the problem. Physical dependence (tolerance or withdrawal symptoms) is still often mistaken as the defining criterion for addiction. We now understand addiction as the compulsive use of a substance that leads to adverse medical or psychosocial consequences. The BRENDA approach evolved because it was apparent that existing treatment models were not fully compatible with the current understanding of addiction, particularly with the use of medications to treat addictions. The following is a brief review of these traditional treatments so that we can define more clearly how the biopsychosocial model of treatment is compatible with many of these traditional approaches. It is not, however, compatible with the moral model that we first discuss.

The Moral Model

Treatment programs are generally not explicitly based on the moral model, but it is the oldest and still most prevalent view of substance addiction and deserves mention here. Essentially, the moral model contends that those who abuse drugs are immoral or lack willpower. Immoral people are thought to yield more easily to temptation, being unable to stop taking drugs or using alcohol. In contrast, normal, decent people put their lives and families first and avoid excessive behaviors.

This approach is highly stigmatizing toward alcoholics and addicts. It puts the blame for the problem squarely on the individual and assumes that all people have equal ability to resist drugs and alcohol. In summary, the reason that addicts and alcoholics become addicted is related to a pervasive immorality.

The implication of a moral model is that addicts and alcoholics do not need treatment; they need to be disciplined. The court system thus becomes the "treatment provider." Yet overwhelming research finds addicts and alcoholics are not "weak willed," and this conclusion is supported by every major medical and psychological society. Despite this, the moral model, still accepted by the general public, is the basis for several interventions aimed at treating alcoholics and addicts. The U.S. Supreme Court has even ruled in a case involving two veterans that their alcohol addictions were a result of "willful misconduct."

Some treatment centers (such as therapeutic communities) aim explicitly at breaking down addicts' personalities, making them admit their wrongs; other programs express disapproval more implicitly. For example, in Alcoholics Anonymous (AA), one step explicitly states that someone in recovery must admit to a defect of character. The sense that addicts and alcoholics are essentially "bad" can be very damaging and, not surprisingly, keep people from seeking treatment. In contrast, the BRENDA model focuses on alleviating, rather than emphasizing, the shame and guilt that accompany the condition.

Pharmacological Determinism

The earliest attempts at looking at drug problems scientifically took a somewhat different tack than the moral model. Rather than blaming the addict for the problem, the cause of addiction was focused on the substance. With opiates, for example, physicians came to believe that after a certain amount of exposure to these drugs, even normal and decent people would lose their will to resist, become enslaved, and would do anything to avoid withdrawal.

An obvious treatment implication of this model was that alcohol and drugs are bad and should be banned. The popularity of pharmacological determinism reached its peak with the Temperance Movement of the early 20th century, in which alcohol in particular was assumed to be an irresistible temptation. However, most Americans did not agree with the vocal segment of the public that saw alcohol as a dangerous drug, and the law establishing Prohibition was repealed when it became obvious that attempts to control alcohol use were failing.

After the repeal of Prohibition, the public's position on alcohol softened but remained harsh with regard to other psychoactive drugs— despite evidence to the contrary showing that like alcohol users, the vast majority of cocaine, heroin, and marijuana users do not become dependent. While pharmacological determinism has waned as a model of addiction, the federal government's "War on Drugs" is clearly an offshoot of this approach.

The Alcoholics Anonymous /Minnesota Model Approach

In 1935, the first widely popular treatment for alcoholism was developed. Created by Bill Wilson and Bob Smith, AA was based on several ideas that became key principles for treatment. Though AA's founders did not espouse some of the concepts, this section describes AA ideology as it is now (Alcoholics Anonymous, 1976). The AA/Minnesota model approach makes the following assumptions:

1. *Alcoholics are essentially different than other drinkers.* AA members believe alcohol itself is not irresistible to everyone, nor is everyone equally likely to be negatively affected by it. Certain people— alcoholics—simply are not able to handle it. After the ideas of alcohol researcher E. M. Jellinek, this model labels this difference as a "disease" or "allergy." Supporters of the model do not believe that alcoholics are less moral than other drinkers; they are simply physiologically incapable of ever drinking moderately. However, they do believe moral remedies are helpful in boosting self-esteem, which is an important part of recovery.

2. *Alcoholics need to feel better about themselves in order to recover, and this cannot happen without an improved spiritual and moral condition.* If alcoholics and addicts are to get better, they have to live a highly moral and spiritual life, which includes making amends for wrongs done and helping other alcoholics recover. These principles are embedded in a "12-step" approach. By taking each of the 12 steps, alcoholics can find a new source of pleasure and purpose to replace the

solace of drinking. Their self-concept and self-esteem improve as they begin to see themselves behaving well.

3. *Alcoholism is a chronic, progressive, and frequently fatal disease if not treated.* Many AA members believe that alcoholism is an integral part of one's personality and may even be genetic. This deeply embedded defect can never be corrected; at best, it can only be arrested by a continued commitment to AA and lifelong abstinence.

Until recently, addiction treatment was based almost entirely on the idea that total abstinence is the only measure of successful treatment. Drug addiction was seen as essentially the same disease as alcoholism and both drug addicts and alcoholics were expected to abstain completely from drugs and alcohol or risk further disease progression. The assumption that the course of addiction is invariably downhill remains prevalent. The American Society of Addiction Medicine still defines alcoholism as a primary, chronic, and often progressive and fatal illness (Morse & Flavin, 1992), even though a great deal of research suggests that many alcoholics do not get progressively worse and some even regain control of their drinking (e.g., Vaillant, 1996; Schukit, Tipp, & Smith, 1997). Treatments based on the learning models of addiction, discussed next, take this into account.

Learning Models

One way to explain the difference between those who can and those who cannot control their use of drugs and alcohol is to look at environmental factors that differentiate people, including variables such as parenting, societal and peer pressure, child abuse, and trauma—in short, anything that might push people toward compulsive use of psychoactive substances and teach them that "drugs are a good thing."

A variety of learning models are used in alcohol dependence treatment (Hester & Miller, 1995). The therapeutic community model views addictive behavior as having developed due to poor parenting and peer role models, and seeks to reparent addicts and teach proper values (Gerstein & Lewin, 1990). Cognitive and behavioral therapies focus on learning to recognize the patterns of thought that lead to excessive drinking and drug use, and replace these behaviors with more healthy coping mechanisms. Learning models assume that addictive behavior is not innate, so some treatments help alcoholics learn to prevent heavy drinking rather than to give up alcohol entirely. While this approach could theoretically be used with illicit drugs as well, most treatment centers avoid doing so because of legal conflicts.

THE BIOPSYCHOSOCIAL APPROACH

The intervention described in this book, referred to as BRENDA, is based on a biopsychosocial model. It incorporates elements of three major models of substance dependence: pharmacological, 12-step, and learning models. From the pharmacological determinist model, it espouses the notion that drugs themselves interact with the brain and may cause changes that reduce an individual's ability to control his or her use. From the 12-step model, it takes the idea that vulnerability to substances varies among individuals and that some people are genetically more vulnerable than others. From the learning model, it draws on the notion that biological changes in vulnerability are not just genetic but may be caused by environmental factors such as child abuse, trauma, or other outside pressures.

People become addicted to substances for a variety of reasons: Some are trying to medicate emotional pain, while others are genetically vulnerable to the pharmacological effects of drugs. In this view, then, addicts or alcoholics are persons who have impaired control over drug and/or alcohol use due to a confluence of factors—most of which are not of their own choosing. Given the complexity of the causes of addiction, it follows that treatment should be individualized to the person seeking help.

Thus, the biopsychosocial model incorporates the use of medications and psychosocial support in an individualized treatment program. This manual was written to address the lack of a formal guide to this kind of treatment. While our research showed that medications are useful in the treatment of addictions, we found resistance in most existing treatment programs to the integration of pharmacotherapy. The use of a medication was seen as a crutch and did not address the "character defect" common to all addicts. We also found that a simple medical approach to addiction—the use of medications without psychosocial support—was often doomed to failure. While the medication may be pharmacologically successful in blocking the drug "high," without psychosocial support, addicts simply stopped taking the medication.

We designed BRENDA as a method to improve patient motivation for treatment and to facilitate recovery using the best available options, including medications. The BRENDA approach has empirical support from research conducted at our center and elsewhere; that is, we have documented the use of BRENDA in a primary care setting, using nurse practitioners and other health care providers (Kaempf, O'Donnell, et al., 1999; Pettinati, Volpicelli, et al., 2000). In addition, the empirical support for the use of brief interventions in which patients receive feedback following a thorough evaluation has been well documented by Miller and his colleagues (Bien, Miller, et al., 1993; Miller, 1998).

A COMPARISON OF THE TYPICAL ALCOHOLICS ANONYMOUS/ MINNESOTA MODEL WITH THE BIOPSYCHOSOCIAL MODEL

In order to fully appreciate how the BRENDA model compares with the most common treatment model (AA or Minnesota model), we present a discussion of the critical differences between these two types of programs. The key points are also summarized in Table 1.1.

Cause of Substance Abuse

According to the AA/Minnesota model, the cause of addiction is primarily a defect in character. The model is not clear as to what causes this defect. It could be genetic predisposition, lack of parental love, abuse, or some spiritual void. In any case, the cause of this personality defect is not considered to be important; rather, these common personality characteristics lead to the behavioral "disease" of addiction in which persons compulsively engage in a variety of addictive behaviors (including but not limited to drugs of abuse), and these compulsive behaviors invariably lead to destruction. While addicted patients often appear to have common personality patterns, prospective studies have failed to demonstrate a unique personality associated with addiction (Schuckit, Klein, et al., 1994). Rather, many of the common personality features observed in addicted patients are a consequence rather than a cause of addiction (Brown, Gleghorn, et al., 1996).

In contrast, the biopsychosocial model assumes that a variety of factors may increase one's risk for addiction, including genetic predispositions, environmental trauma, social learning, and the interaction of

TABLE 1.1. A Comparison of the BRENDA and AA/Minnesota Models

	BRENDA model	AA/Minnesota model
Cause of substance abuse	Biopsychosocial	Disease/character defect
Level of care	Ambulatory	Inpatient intensive
Duration of treatment	Long-term with follow-ups	Acute with AA aftercare
Use of medications	Extensive	Limited
Practitioners	Various—team approach	Drug and alcohol counselors
View of relapse	Biopsychosocial factors, learning opportunities	Person not "working the program," back to Step 1
Desired outcome	Improved functioning	Total abstinence
Research support	Extensive—empirically based	Limited
Psychosocial support	BRENDA approach	Requires AA/group therapy

these biopsychosocial factors. No assumption is made that an addictive personality exists or that addicted individuals have inherently different personalities than others. Social attitudes toward addiction, particularly the moral perspective, often engender feelings of guilt and shame, which may inadvertently lead to denial, lying, and avoidance.

Level of Care

The typical addiction treatment program refers persons for inpatient detoxification and a 28-day rehabilitation. There are no good scientific data to support the use of inpatient over outpatient care, but inpatient care does get the addict away from his or her environment and in some cases helps the family cope with a crisis that may have been precipitated by alcohol or other drug abuse. With the advent of managed care, the use of inpatient programs is now less common, and less restrictive environments, such as intensive outpatient, day treatment, or residential treatment programs, offer some cost advantages. In any case, the basic assumption is that intensive and frequent contact needs to be established to initiate abstinence. Given the high rate of relapse when a patient is discharged from an intensive program and the high cost to provide daily treatment, it is time to rethink the notion that inpatient treatment is a necessary option for most addicts.

The assumption of the biopsychosocial model presented here is that treatment needs to be individualized for the needs of the patient. While some patients are truly in a medical, emotional, or social crisis, the vast majority of patients need a program that helps them learn to cope with their addiction. Research generally shows that ambulatory detoxification programs and day treatment rehabilitation programs are as effective and much less expensive than inpatient programs (Hayashida, Alterman, et al., 1989).

Treatment and Its Duration

The AA/Minnesota model assumes that addiction is caused by a character defect. Thus, a healthy, drug-free lifestyle will result only by correcting that defect of character. This is accomplished by acknowledging the problem, working the 12 steps, relying on social supports, and turning one's will and life over to a higher power that will then remove these defects of character. The duration of professional treatment is relatively brief, since the goal is to get the patient to acknowledge the problem, safely detoxify from alcohol or other drugs, and then accept referral to AA or other 12-step support groups. The role of the professional counselor is limited to the early stages of recovery.

In contrast, the biopsychosocial approach assumes that a variety of biological, psychological, and social factors all contribute to the risk for addiction, and even after the patient is no longer using alcohol or drugs, successful treatment needs to address these risk factors. For example, a significant percentage of patients with addiction will have comorbid psychiatric disorders, and successful treatment involves addressing these issues as well as drug use. Addiction is viewed as a chronic disorder, not unlike diabetes or hypertension. Even when the acute problem is stabilized, long-term follow-up is required to reduce risk factors for an exacerbation of symptoms, to attend to other co-occurring problems, and to maintain a relationship with a health care provider to monitor progress and reduce the severity of relapse should it occur.

Use of Medications

If addiction is caused by a defect of character, then there is limited rationale for the use of medications to treat addictions. Rather, medications, except for the early detoxification phase of treatment, are seen as a crutch and can inhibit personal growth.

In contrast, from a biopsychosocial perspective, medications can have an important role in reducing the biological underpinnings of addiction and reduce alcohol and drug craving, and the possibility of relapse by treating co-occurring medical or psychiatric conditions that could lead to relapse, such as chronic pain syndromes, depression, and anxiety disorders.

Practitioners

Typically, AA/Minnesota model programs use as the primary treatment providers addiction counselors, who often have personal experience with addiction. The use of counselors who themselves have participated in AA makes sense if the assumption is that the goal of treatment is to help patients realize their problem and facilitate referral to self-help programs.

In contrast, a biopsychosocial model employs a variety of treatment providers to address the many medical, psychological, and social complications resulting from addiction and the biopsychosocial factors that may increase the risk for relapse. Addiction counselors remain a part of the team of health care professionals but are aided by health care professionals from other disciplines.

As mentioned earlier, the use of medications is an integral part of treatment, so medical health care providers are needed to prescribe and monitor medications. In addition, mental health care providers are often called upon to address co-occurring behavioral and emotional disorders. Finally, family and couple therapists also have an important role in treatment, particularly in helping patients cope effectively with relationship issues, without the use of alcohol or other drugs.

View of Relapse

In the view of the AA/Minnesota model, relapse is a consequence of not actively working the 12 steps. When relapse occurs, persons begin again at Step 1, having "lost" credit for all the sober time they accumulated before the relapse.

In contrast, the biopsychosocial model looks at the cause of relapse in terms of the factors that predispose persons to become addicted in the first place. Given addiction's chronic nature, relapses are a common occurrence and, while not a cause for celebration, they are not a reason for despair. Often, one can learn valuable lessons from a relapse, and the treatment plan can incorporate changes that further improve the treatment outcome.

Desired Outcome

In an AA/Minnesota model approach, the only possible desired outcome for an addict is complete and lifelong abstinence. Attention is given primarily to any alcohol or psychoactive drug use, with less emphasis on other compulsive behaviors such as overeating, gambling, and so on. Ironically, little attention is paid to one of the most addictive substances, nicotine, which is responsible for more drug-related fatalities in the United States than all other abusive drugs combined.

In contrast, the biopsychosocial model is primarily interested in levels of physical, emotional, and social health. While abstinence is typically the preferred outcome, there is room for individual differences in treatment. Alcohol and drug use is viewed in the context of overall health. Not only is the absence of alcohol and drug abuse desired, but also a physically and emotionally healthy functioning person is the desired outcome.

Research Support

The AA/Minnesota model is based on the experience of millions of people who have tried this approach. Little scientific research demonstrates its effectiveness over some control condition, but two recent, large, multicentered clinical trials demonstrate that the AA philosophy, when administered in a well-controlled setting with experienced addiction counselors, leads to outcomes as good or better than other psychosocial approaches (Match Group, 1997; Crits-Christoph, Siqueland, et al., 1999).

The biopsychosocial model is based on the past quarter century of research conducted at addiction research centers in the United States and elsewhere (Woody, McLellan, et al., 1990; McLellan, Arndt, et al., 1993; O'Brien, 1997; Volpicelli, Rhines, et al., 1997). Since the assumption is that research studies help to discover truths about addic-

tion, the biopsychosocial approach is constantly evolving as new research leads to advances in our understanding and treatment.

Psychosocial Support

The AA/Minnesota model requires everyone to adhere to the 12-step
approach to treatment. While it is stated that one can take from the program what works for him or her, it is assumed that acceptance of the entire program leads to the best results.

Within the biopsychosocial approach, a variety of psychosocial
options are given to patients, including referrals to self-help groups
such as AA. The program is a collaboration between the patient, health
care provider, and a team of other health care providers that facilitate
various aspects of treatment.

In the next chapter we present an overview of the elements of the
BRENDA model and demonstrate a typical treatment encounter.

▬

CHAPTER 2

Managing Addiction Treatment Using the BRENDA Approach

BRENDA is a patient-centered model. Unlike most treatment models that mandate coverage of particular issues at particular times, the content and timing of the six stages of BRENDA are solely dependent on the patient's progress through the model; that is, all six stages of BRENDA could be approached in one session, or any given session might focus on only one of the six stages. In general, however, the stages follow the sequence in the acronym, BRENDA.

The BRENDA method is based on the biopsychosocial model of addiction and so begins with a thorough biopsychosocial assessment of complications arising from excessive alcohol drinking or other drug use. Based on the biopsychosocial assessment, treatment recommendations use a variety of individualized medical and psychosocial interventions for the patient.

Most treatment programs assume their responsibility ends with making an accurate assessment of substance abuse and then giving direct advice for treatment. We feel that this is not enough. It is the responsibility of the treatment provider to help motivate patients to engage and remain in treatment, and to comply with the treatment recommendations, including compliance with taking prescribed medications. The six BRENDA stages are designed to improve the motivation to change and to enhance treatment and medication adherence primarily by establishing a collaborative therapeutic alliance between the patient and practitioner. This includes a report back to the patient in a nonjudgmental fashion of the results of the biopsychosocial evaluation, an empathetic understanding of the problem from the patient's perspective, and a special emphasis on reviewing the needs and desired outcomes for each individual patient. When treatment recommendations are given to a patient within the context of an understanding, therapeutic relationship, the chance that a patient will carry through with the recommendations is improved. In contrast to most existing treatment programs, failure to follow through or accept treatment recommendations is not seen as a failure on the patient's part, but rather reflects a mismatch in the recommendations given by the health care provider and the needs or abilities of the patient.

COMPONENTS OF THE BRENDA APPROACH

The following six stages summarize the BRENDA approach. The use of the acronym BRENDA provides an easy way to remember the sequence of steps:

B—Biopsychosocial evaluation
R—Report to the patient on assessment
E—Empathetic understanding of the patient's problem
N—Needs expressed by the patient that should be addressed
D—Direct advice on how to meet those needs
A—Assessing responses/behaviors of the patient to advice and adjusting treatment recommendations

We discuss each of the six stages in more detail throughout the manual, but first we present an overview of the BRENDA method and the rationale for each stage.

Biopsychosocial Evaluation

The biopsychosocial evaluation (**B**) is typically the initial step. The BRENDA approach is distinguished from other treatment approaches in that an addiction history is integrated with a thorough medical and psychosocial evaluation. The attention to the medical history helps to identify medical complications at an early stage, while treatment can be less intensive and more effective. For example, elevations in liver enzymes may be a warning sign of the potential for serious liver infections or cirrhosis. In addition, the psychosocial evaluation can help to uncover serious psychological or psychiatric disorders that are common in addicts. Furthermore, when these co-occurring psychological or psychiatric disorders are effectively treated, addiction treatment outcomes may be improved (Woody, McLellan, et al., 1990; Kranzler, Burleson, et al., 1994).

Report to the Patient

Next, the results of the biopsychosocial evaluation are presented to the patient. When combined with empathy (see below), feedback in the form of a report (**R**) helps to establish a collaborative relationship between the patient and practitioner, and is also an important factor in motivating behavioral changes. For example, giving patients feedback about their abnormally elevated liver enzymes and a recommendation to cut back on drinking can have a dramatic effect in reducing excessive alcohol consumption.

Empathetic Understanding

Empathy (**E**) is a part of each of the stages in the BRENDA method but is particularly important following the presentation of the report. Research shows that people who feel understood are more likely to accept recommendations from others. At this point, some patients may refute the report—"I am not an alcoholic, and I don't think that my side is tender from liver problems." Rather than debate or nag patients, it is important to understand their perspective and how they feel about the report just presented, which may elicit fear, denial, hopelessness, or shame. Whatever the feeling, it is important to acknowledge and understand the affect and thoughts that accompany the presentation of the biopsychosocial evaluation.

Needs Expressed by the Patient

After one gains an empathetic understanding of the addiction problem, one can accurately assess the needs (**N**) and goals of the patient. These needs, as expressed by the patient, may not be the same as those that family members or a treatment provider have for the patient. So, for example, someone who has marital problems, psychological distress, and liver disease may need marital therapy from the spouse's perspective, or psychological counseling from a therapist's perspective, but from the patient's own perspective, the problem that is causing the most concern is elevations in his or her liver enzymes. Rather than try to convince patients of what their needs should be, a treatment provider has a responsibility to the patient's own priorities and needs for treatment. This approach contrasts sharply with other models of addiction treatment, where the task of the treatment provider is to convince the patient to change his or her behavior or wait until he or she is ready to change, often after "hitting rock bottom." In the BRENDA model, the therapist works collaboratively with patients to identify their needs so that they can move toward recovery.

Direct Advice

After the patient's needs are uncovered and mutually agreed upon by therapist and patient, the treatment provider then presents direct advice (**D**) and recommendations for treatment options. This advice should specifically address the patient's needs. For example, if a patient expresses a need to reduce liver toxicity, then a program of abstinence and perhaps medications that control excessive drinking would be the recommendation. If a patient does not identify marital satisfaction as an important need at that time, it is unlikely that a recommendation for family counseling would be followed. However, a seed may be planted: Should the marital problems get worse or not improve over a period of time, this matter would need to be readdressed.

Assess Patient Responses

The final stage in the BRENDA approach is to assess (**A**) the patient's behavioral response to the direct advice. This assessment takes place after the provider presents the treatment recommendations. For example, you may recommend that patients with liver disease obtain additional blood work to rule out hepatitis C, or you may suggest a graduated schedule for maintaining periods of alcohol abstinence. You then assess the patient's reactions both immediately and in the following session. A patient may react by agreeing to the blood tests but not want to become completely abstinent. At the next visit, you may even discover that the patient failed to get his or her blood tested. Here, the BRENDA approach most clearly differs from other approaches. Rather than assume the patient is not ready for treatment or is in denial, the reasons for his or her objections need to be explored. Perhaps, the patient does not understand the evidence that went into the recommendation. In this case, the health care provider can review the results of the blood tests and their significance, explaining to the patient, "Your liver enzyme results are dangerously high and this could intensify if you continue to drink. If you have hepatitis C, the liver damage can occur even more rapidly." The treatment provider can also try to understand from the patient's perspective why he or she wants to continue to drink. It may be that he or she is unable to comply with the recommendation: "I could never completely give up alcohol." In addition, perhaps the person does not believe complete abstinence is necessary: "What if I just cut down on my drinking?" Finally, if the patient replies, "It's not that bad yet. I have a stronger need to drink than to deal with a problem that does not bother me so much," the health care provider can reassess the situation if the patient really sees a need to cope with liver disease.

As this example shows, the first four stages, "B-R-E-N," provide the foundation for direct and specific recommendations. If the patient objects to the therapist's recommendations, then perhaps new recommendations can be offered that can be agreed upon. For example, the treatment provider and patient may agree that if the patient can limit him- or herself to three or fewer drinks per day and a retest of the liver enzymes shows an improvement, then the recommendation for complete abstinence can be modified.

The assessment stage in the BRENDA approach extends beyond a treatment session and becomes a tool to change dynamically the treatment recommendations over time. For example, if the patient agreed to try to limit his or her drinking but had several episodes of excessive drinking between treatment visits, then the direct advice may again be to consider complete abstinence as a goal.

Each of the BRENDA stages outlined earlier is designed to improve retention in treatment and compliance with treatment recommendations. Since the treatment recommendations are based on specific medical or psychosocial problems that are unique to the patient and are a collaborative effort between the treatment provider and patient, many of the barriers to treatment compliance are broken down. The rationale for these six stages comes from research derived from the stages of change concept and the use of motivational interviewing to affect behavioral changes.

Integration of BRENDA with Stages of Change and Motivational Interviewing

The BRENDA approach to addiction treatment assumes that all addicted patients are not at the same level of motivation to change their behavior. Some people may not believe their alcohol or drug use is a problem; others may be unsure if their drug use is a problem; and still others may be fairly certain they want to change their behavior but are unsure what to do. An approach that fails to take into account the motivational state of the addicted person is likely to lead to a poor outcome or "resistance."

An excellent tool for tailoring interventions to an individual's substance dependence problems is the "stages of change" model developed by Prochaska and colleagues (Prochaska, DiClemente, et al., 1992). There are six stages of change: precontemplation, contemplation, preparation, action, maintenance, and relapse. Different motivational strategies are useful in each stage, and the goal of recovery is to move patients toward the "action" and "maintenance" stages. These stages are not unique to substance dependence treatment. They can be applied to any human activity in which a change in behavior is attempted, for example, starting an exercise or nutritional program. Providers may come into contact with addicted patients in any of the stages of change and get a sense of patients' stage of change by their reaction to the report of the biopsychosocial evaluation.

Precontemplators are unaware that they have a problem and typically are unmotivated to change or seek treatment. Also, in many cases, they are not even defensive about the idea of having a problem or needing treatment because they believe the problem does not pertain to them. Precontemplators, with respect to addiction problems, are more likely seen among patients seeking treatment for medical problems in primary care settings than among those seeking treatment for an alcohol or drug problem in specialized addiction programs. To motivate precontemplators for addiction treatment, you need to provide concrete evidence of the possibility that their drinking or drug use may be harmful and help them recognize that they are capable of changing it.

Contemplators tend at least to have thought about the possibility that they might have a problem. However, they have not yet decided whether to accept the idea or to do anything to change their behavior. They are typically ambivalent (i.e., unsure if the evidence necessitates change). They are also afraid that to try to change and fail would be too great a blow to their self-esteem. To motivate contemplators, you try to help them understand that change is necessary, and that they are capable of changing. For contemplators, a kind of cost–benefit analysis is taking place. The report just presented can give weight to the costs of addiction, but to tip the scales in favor of taking action, you should give special attention to an understanding of the patient's own reasons for treating the addiction: the Needs assessment.

Persons in the third stage, *preparation*, have decided that they have a problem and need to take action. Miller describes this phase as a brief window of opportunity: It opens for a time, but if the person does not have access to what he or she needs in order to get better, it closes and the change process is aborted. Keep in mind that you may need to go beyond your own services in assisting the patient to change. In these cases, you should be proactive about introducing the patient to a variety of treatment options that you feel would be useful to the patient.

In the *action* stage, persons choose a change strategy and act on it. Here, again, patients need encouragement and support. A most important aspect in this stage is to convey continually to patients that you are optimistic about their recovery and to help patients believe in their ability to recover.

Finally, the *maintenance* stage can be a difficult phase for many patients, and when it occurs, the treatment may vary greatly from patient to patient. As Mark Twain said about cigarettes, "Quitting is easy, I've done it a thousand times." However, maintaining abstinence is difficult, and treatment at this point needs to focus directly on helping the patient stay abstinent. In BRENDA, patients in the maintenance stage should rapidly cycle through the six BRENDA stages. There need to be frequent reviews of the results of the Biopsychosocial assessment of how things were for the patient at treatment entry, how they are now, and why they are better. Patient reactions to this line of discussion are most important and will help you determine their unique Needs at this phase in the treatment. Direct advice can be adjusted accordingly, so that future Assessment shows continued progress and treatment adherence.

Relapse, of course, is what happens when the plan developed for maintenance fails and the patient returns to pretreatment levels of drinking or drug use. Relapse should not be viewed as a failure of treatment as a whole, but rather as failure only of the specific plan. It is an event to learn from and a possible spur for devising a better plan and rapid return to the maintenance stage.

INTEGRATION OF STAGES OF CHANGE AND TREATMENT COMPLIANCE

The best predictor of treatment compliance is motivation to change. Those who adhere most to treatment recommendations and stay in treatment are most likely to have the best outcomes. For this reason, an important component of any treatment program, particularly those that use medications as part of treatment, is enhancement of the patient's motivation to change.

Research on Medication Compliance

Recent studies have found that patients who take naltrexone as prescribed show a markedly lower relapse rate than those taking a placebo. Approximately 50% of patients on placebo compared to 25% on naltrexone relapsed to heavy drinking in the first 3 months of treatment (Volpicelli, Rhines, et al., 1997). Also, among those who impulsively took a drink, 90% of patients on placebo compared to 40% on naltrexone relapsed (Volpicelli, Rhines, et al., 1997). In patients who did not take all of their prescribed naltrexone, the difference in relapse rates between the naltrexone and the placebo group was not statistically significant. In summary, to maximize the effectiveness of naltrexone, be sure to provide an intervention, for example, BRENDA, to ensure medication compliance.

While a small percentage of patients adhering to a medication regimen of naltrexone, experience uncomfortable side effects such as tiredness, anxiety, nausea, and vomiting, this is not the only factor in predicting who skips doses or stops taking the medication altogether. Other factors include patient ambivalence about giving up alcohol and difficulty in the patient–provider relationship (Volpicelli, Rhines, et al., 1997).

How BRENDA Addresses Denial of Disorder

Patients who do not adhere to treatment recommendations are often said to be in denial about their alcohol or other drug problem. "Denial," or noncompliance, is not the sole preserve of those with drug and alcohol problems. It is a major contributor to treatment noncompliance in almost every aspect of medicine. In a number of treatable, chronic conditions (including bipolar disorder, hypertension, diabetes, and many other conditions), research has identified denial as a "high risk" factor in predicting treatment noncompliance. Reports abound on the patient's refusal to accept the fact that he or she has a chronic illness or to believe that the condition is "so bad" that medication is necessary. Patients may not always verbalize this sort of thinking. However, patients who do not accept that medication is needed and helpful frequently will not take it.

An important part of dealing with denial, then, is to provide the patient with full knowledge of his or her condition and its treatment. This is a natural part of BRENDA, when results of the **R**eport are discussed initially and then referred to from time to time over the course of the BRENDA visits. Clinicians should also discuss fears patients may have about taking medications for any prolonged period of time. It is important to stress that the medication being prescribed is safe and generally well tolerated.

How BRENDA Builds a Relationship between Clinician and Patient

Another common reason for medication noncompliance is difficulty in the relationship between the patient and the clinician. There are frequently two factors at work: The first is the patient's sense of distrust of authority, which results in a power struggle; the second is the patient's skepticism that medication will help.

Since patients with substance dependence are frequently told what to do and how bad their problems are, it is particularly important to avoid getting into a power struggle. The key is to listen to the patient so you can develop **E**mpathetic understanding, which in turn will foster strong alliance with the patient. In order to get optimum medication compliance, you need to be sure that patients see you as being on their side rather than trying to force something on them that they do not want and do not see as helpful to them.

Pay attention to the patient's Needs with regard to treatment. Once you know these, you can then use them to motivate patients to take medication. If, for example, someone believes that avoiding medical problems is the most important reason he or she needs to stop drinking, then emphasize how the medication will help in his or her quest for health. If, on the other hand, the patient could care less about health effects and instead cares more about work performance, emphasize how the medication, by helping prevent relapse, will help him or her perform better on the job.

Additional problems that may arise in the patient and clinician relationship include patient skepticism about the efficacy of the medication. To avoid this, be sure that you express confidence in any treatment you provide. Be positive and share important known facts or research on the medication with the patient, letting him or her know that you have great reason to think this will be helpful. See Appendix B for an overview or consult Berg, Pettinatti, et al. (1996) for facts on naltrexone.

OVERVIEW OF THE COURSE OF TREATMENT: HOW THE COMPONENTS WORK TOGETHER

Addiction treatment consists of three major stages: (1) initiating treatment, (2) detoxification and stabilization, and (3) recovery. While there is no set formula for the duration and intensity of treatment, the following example is fairly typical as someone goes through the various stages of treatment.

Initiation of Treatment

Perhaps the most difficult and challenging stage of treatment is the initiation stage, when people are at various levels of readiness to enter into treatment. The BRENDA approach is useful in this stage of treatment, when someone may come to the attention of a health care provider for some perceived nonaddiction problem such as stomach pains or symptoms of depression. When such patients present for treatment, they may not be aware or ready to accept that they have an alcohol or drug problem. Components of the BRENDA approach have been used successfully in brief interventions that have been published in the literature

(Miller, Benefield, et al., 1993). For example, an initial evaluation followed by giving patients feedback or a report of their addiction-related problems has been shown to be as effective as the Minnesota model inpatient treatments in several empirical studies (Hester & Miller, 1995). The BRENDA approach can be used as a brief intervention to initiate treatment, as illustrated in the following example:

> James, a 38-year-old, employed postal worker was seen by his local primary care physician, Dr. K, because of intermittent abdominal pain. Dr. K did a physical exam after he administered an alcohol screening instrument, the CAGE questionnaire. At the first interview, James's physician reviewed the results of the CAGE questionnaire and his physical exam finding of an enlarged, tender liver.
>
> He then conducted a brief substance abuse history. James denied that he was using any nonprescription drugs or that he drank excessively. He did admit that he binged on alcohol most weekends and would show up at work on Mondays with a severe hangover. He also admitted that after work most days, he "would have a couple of drinks with his friends" before returning home (**B**). In a nonjudgmental fashion, Dr. K suggested that James might have an alcohol problem (**R**). James immediately reacted with disbelief, claiming, "I'm no alcoholic." Dr. K asked how James defined an alcoholic, and James said, "An alcoholic is someone who can't hold a job and gets drunk every day." Dr. K replied, "I can see why you do not believe you are an alcoholic by that definition." Dr. K then suggested that an alcohol problem was just one of several possible explanations for the abdominal pain (**E**). James said that all he needed was something to take away his abdominal pain, and Dr. K agreed that this was his primary concern as well (**N**). Dr. K suggested that in order to diagnose the cause of the abdominal pain, he needed to obtain some blood tests for hepatitis screening and liver function (**D**). Dr. K did not argue with James but suggested that they meet again in a few days to see if the abdominal pain was still present, and to review the laboratory data. James agreed to meet again (**A**). At the next appointment a few days later, as Dr. K reviewed the results of the abnormally high liver enzyme results, James decided he wanted to do something to stop his problem with alcohol.

If a brief intervention does not help a patient initiate treatment, then you should set up a follow-up visit in a month or so to reassess the person's readiness to change. If the person is still not ready to initiate treatment, you can conduct follow-up evaluations at periodic intervals (three to four times per year) to assess whether the addiction has progressed, and whether the person is ready to initiate treatment.

Detoxification/Stabilization

Once patients decide that they would like to begin treatment, they need to be evaluated for the possibility of medical detoxification from alcohol or other drugs. Additionally, any other medical or psychosocial emergent problems should be assessed and appropriate treatment options offered to help stabilize the patient. The biopsychosocial evaluation during this stage of treatment should focus on ruling out medical or psychiatric emergencies that would necessitate an inpatient admission. The vast majority of addicts (85%) can safely and effectively complete alcohol detoxification in an outpatient setting. The aggressive use of ambulatory treatment offers significant cost savings without sacrificing safety or efficacy (Hayashida, Alterman, et al., 1989).

Typically, detoxification occurs over a 1- to 2-week period of brief (15 to 30 minutes) daily visits with a medical health care provider to monitor withdrawal symptoms and to prescribe medications to relieve withdrawal symptoms. The specific medications to treat withdrawal depend on the drug of abuse and severity of withdrawal symptoms. Typically, when a drug is abruptly stopped, the body responds by overreacting in the opposite direction to the drug of abuse. For example, sedative abuse leads to hyperactive physiological responses. Medications that reduce withdrawal symptoms can help people safely stop using alcohol and other drugs. A fairly typical detoxification follows:

> Once James agreed to begin treatment, Dr. K evaluated his need for detoxification. The history and physical exam revealed that James had symptoms of alcohol withdrawal, so he was given a prescription for Serax (oxazepam) and vitamins, and was told to return every day for the next 5 days. During this time, Dr. K continued to collect data on the severity of withdrawal symptoms and was able to show James his progress as measured by an alcohol withdrawal scale. Even in these relatively brief sessions Dr. K used the BRENDA method continually to provide a report on James's progress. James felt that Dr. K understood his need to

sleep and avoid feelings of anxiousness about giving up alcohol. Dr. K's treatment recommendations reflected James's need to avoid the unpleasant alcohol withdrawal symptoms. As a result, James enthusiastically supported the treatment recommendations by taking the medications as prescribed and attending all the follow-up visits.

The detoxification stage is quite variable in its intensity and duration depending on the initial severity of the presenting problems and the patient's response during treatment. At one extreme, someone who has refrained from drug or alcohol use for several days before initiating treatment, has minimal withdrawal symptoms, has no medical or psychiatric emergencies, and has a stable social situation (e.g., a place to live) may quickly pass through this stage into the recovery stage. In contrast, other people who are medically unstable (e.g., impending delirium tremens, DTs), have severe emotional distress (e.g., suicidal thoughts), or have an unstable social support (e.g., were just kicked out of the house) may need more intensive attention during this stage. Once these emergent problems are stabilized, the third stage of treatment may commence.

Recovery Stage

The recovery stage can be divided into two phases presented as the early and later stages. Again, there is no fixed number or duration of sessions. A typical patient going through BRENDA treatment will meet with a health care provider in an outpatient setting once a week for between 20 and 40 minutes the first 3 months of treatment (early phase), then for 12 biweekly sessions (later phase). Following a treatment episode, we suggest that visits continue to be scheduled at monthly intervals for another 6 months. This extends a treatment episode to 12 months, then every 3 to 4 months, follow-up visits are scheduled to monitor progress. The duration of treatment, substantially longer than typical treatment programs, is more realistic in obtaining and sustaining long-term recovery. Treatment sessions occur in an outpatient setting, allowing the patient to maintain other social responsibilities such as work or taking care of children. During this time, referrals to other health care providers are often made to complement treatment. In sub-

sequent chapters, we review the focus and goals of the various phases
of treatment and present illustrative cases.

Following detoxification, James was prescribed a medication, naltrexone, to help control alcohol craving and reduce his chances of
relapse. James was seen every week by Dr. K for the first 12 weeks
of treatment and was compliant with all treatment recommendations, including taking all his medications. While James reported
little alcohol craving and no drinking, Dr. K noticed that James expressed concern that his relationship with his girlfriend was not
going well. He recommended that James and his girlfriend see a
couple therapist, Jan, to help improve their relationship. James and
his girlfriend then met with Jan for weekly sessions over the
course of 6 months. In addition to his sessions with Jan, James
continued to see Dr. K, who reminded James to take his medications and reinforced the notion that the combination of medications and psychosocial support was having a large impact on his
recovery. After the first 12 weeks, sessions with Dr. K were reduced to every other week for medication management for the next
3 months.

Despite the couple therapy sessions, James and his girlfriend
split up 6 months into treatment. But James continues to see the
therapist individually. The psychosocial aspects of James's drinking became more apparent as James opened up about his relationship difficulties. During this phase of treatment, the focus of therapy was more related to social relationships, particularly his
relationship with women, and generally learning to cope with life
challenges without the use of alcohol or drugs. Remaining abstinent from alcohol, James noted a void in his life. With the therapist, James began to explore ways to meet women and to understand why his previous relationships never progressed beyond a
superficial stage. At this point, James found himself discussing
deep personal issues with the therapist in a way that surprised him.
He trusted the therapist and felt an unconditional acceptance and
understanding that allowed him to open up about his conflicted relationships with his parents.

James remained on naltrexone for a total of 9 months. During
this time, he discovered he missed drinking less and less. His liver
enzymes returned to normal and his abdominal pain vanished. In
contrast to other programs in which medical and psychosocial care
are fragmented or perhaps even at odds with one another, James

felt that both his therapist and Dr. K were working together in his best interest.

Often, patients who have been sober for 6 to 9 months may find that medications such as naltrexone can be safely discontinued. In some cases, however, long-term use of medications may be helpful. As in other chronic diseases, long-term follow-up is important to warn of potential clinical deterioration.

On the advice of Dr. K, James stopped the naltrexone after being sober for 9 months. For James, the next 6 months of treatment helped create important changes in his social relationships. He began to date a woman who knew about his addiction to alcohol yet was quite supportive of his recovery. At work, James received a promotion to supervisor and in general felt more content and happy than at any time in his life. He continued to see his therapist at monthly intervals for a year, and then at 4-month intervals to monitor progress. Now, 4 years later, James is married, and except for an alcohol slip and near relapse 2 years ago, he continues to feel happy and productive.

As this example shows, there are a number of specific things that a professional must know and be able to perform in order to implement BRENDA, including:

- Accurately understanding the difference between recreational use of a drug and addiction.
- Conducting a comprehensive biopsychosocial addiction evaluation.
- Having a nonjudgmental approach toward obtaining information from individuals presenting for treatment.
- Monitoring progress in treatment.
- Working together with other health care professionals to better coordinate a comprehensive treatment program.

Each of these is discussed as the chapters that follow describe in detail the six BRENDA stages. Table 2.1 lays out the steps and their related tasks. In Chapter 3, we further discuss not only current understanding of addiction and how it can be distinguished from recreational substance use but also how to conduct a **B**iopsychosocial addiction evalua-

TABLE 2.1. The BRENDA Method

B   Biopsychosocial evaluation
Biological and medical assessment
Psychological assessment
Social assessment

R   Report
Formulate patient profile based on evaluation
Report evaluation results to patient
Assess patient reactions to report/assess stage of change

E   Empathy
Listen to understand the patient's emotional reaction to report
Express understanding of the patient's emotional reaction given his or her
assumptions
Challenge negative assumptions underlying the patient's distress

N   Needs
Immediate, basic health and safety needs
Patient needs from biopsychosocial deficits
Patient priorities

D   Direct advice
Match patient needs to available resources
Present a menu of treatment options; emphasize patient choice
Point out how options help achieve patient priorities

A   Assess patient reactions to advice/adjust advice
Reassess biopsychosocial status and give positive feedback
Compare patient status with patient goal for recovery
Assess whether the patient is following up on direct advice and treatment
recommendations
Link patient actions (inaction) on advice to changes in biopsychosocial
status; adjust advice if needed

tion. Chapter 4 covers how to prepare and present the Report of the assessment to the patient. Chapters 5, 6, 7, and 8 detail how to carry out the remaining steps: Empathy, Needs identification, Direct advice, and Assessment, including monitoring treatment progress. Chapter 9 discusses pharmacotherapy and issues around medication compliance. Chapters 10 and 11 discuss how the BRENDA approach can be adapted to issues in the early and later stages of recovery. Chapters 12, 13, and

14 present three case examples of how a series of BRENDA visits might be structured. Appendix A provides several useful instruments to identify people with alcohol and other drug problems and a brief instrument to measure psychological distress. Appendix B provides detailed information on prescribing naltrexone, a medication approved by the U.S. Food and Drug Administration for treating alcohol dependence.

CHAPTER 3

▬▬▬

Biopsychosocial Assessment

How to Conduct It

Bill, a 57-year-old corporate CEO, has three children, one from a previous marriage, who remains with his first wife, and two with his second wife. He has come for a physical exam after several years of going without medical care ("too busy") in order to "get his wife off his back."

Alissa, a 25-year-old, single mother of two on public assistance, presents for treatment to a mental health clinic with recurrent suicidal thoughts. She seems extremely thin and jittery, and cannot sit still during the interview.

Stephen, 34, a construction worker, has just broken his leg in an on-the-job accident. During his evaluation by the company nurse, he was found to be intoxicated and referred to the Employee Assistance Program (EAP) addiction counselor.

CROSSING THE LINE: SCREENING FOR ADDICTION

None of these patients has sought treatment for substance dependence, yet each exhibits potential warning signs of a drug or alcohol problem.

How do we know when a person has crossed the line from recreational drug use to addiction? Our understanding of addiction has radically changed in the past two decades. Whereas addiction was once thought to be the same as physical dependence on a drug, we now understand addiction in terms of compulsive use of alcohol or drugs leading to a variety of medical and psychosocial consequences. The emphasis on the medical and psychosocial consequences that result from compulsive use of alcohol or other drugs naturally leads to our modern concept of addiction as a biopsychosocial disorder.

Historically, addiction was defined in physical terms and focused on drug tolerance and withdrawal symptoms. The term "physical dependence" is still often used synonymously with addiction, but physical dependence, or physiological adaptation, is not the same as addiction. Consider the following example: A patient who has just undergone abdominal surgery has been taking morphine daily for several days for pain relief. If she abruptly stops taking the morphine, she experiences withdrawal symptoms. Yet as long as she continues her pain medication, she experiences no cravings, and she never uses more morphine than prescribed by her doctor. In fact, the doctor has given her control over the amount of morphine she needs to treat her pain and, as a result, she can gradually reduce her dose over time with minimal discomfort. She is not addicted to morphine, and in fact, the morphine improves her rate of recovery from the surgery.

Addiction is not simply using a lot of a drug. Often, in health care settings, patients are asked about the quantity and frequency of their drinking, but this can be a particularly poor way to assess addiction. For example, patient A has a drink every day after work and on weekends drinks large quantities of alcohol with his friends and at social functions. Yet patient A can limit his drinking so as not to interfere with his health, work, or social life. He can enjoy a beer, but when he is the designated driver, he can easily limit himself to one beer on those evenings. In contrast, patient B drinks much less frequently than patient A, but when he drinks, he finds that once he begins drinking, he binges until he becomes grossly intoxicated and often engages in reckless behavior such as drunk driving. We would define patient B as addicted but not patient A even though patient A has more total drinks in a month than patient B.

We now understand addiction as the compulsive use of a substance that leads to adverse medical or psychosocial consequences. This compulsive use is a manifestation of impaired control over the substance and is experienced by addicts as an increased need for the drug the more they use it. There is an old Asian proverb that clearly describes addiction: "First the man takes a drink, then the drink takes a drink, and then the drink takes the man." The line between being a recreational user of a drug and being at risk for addiction is crossed when one has difficulty controlling his or her drug use. For example, it is often remarked that "one drink is too many, while 100 drinks are not enough." As is recognized in most addiction recovery programs, this notion of impaired control is the hallmark of addiction. With impaired control, other important priorities lose out to the compulsion to drink, smoke, or inject the drug.

Several important features mark substance addiction:

- The person's control over drinking or drug intake is impaired, and he or she finds it difficult or impossible to cut back or stop using substances.
- The substance use has reduced the person's quality of life and his or her world has become centered on using substances. The person continues to use alcohol or drugs despite repeated, adverse drinking or drug-related consequences (e.g., medical problems, arrests for driving under the influence [DUI], missed days at work, family fights).
- The person uses alcohol or drugs to relieve or avoid withdrawal symptoms or drug craving. This addictive cycle creates a pattern in which drug use begets more drug use.

The modern definition of addiction requires more than simply asking how much alcohol is consumed or if one is using a psychoactive drug. Rather, screening should emphasize drug use that is compulsive (impaired control), leads to biopsychosocial problems, and creates a vicious cycle in which drug use begets more drug use.

APPROACH TO ASSESSMENT

Special Issues in the Initial Presentation for Treatment

The initial assessment should be a routine part of the evaluation of any patient who presents with a medical or psychological problem. Given the high rates of addiction in virtually all treatment settings, it is important to screen for addiction in any medical or mental health care setting. There is no excuse for the low rates of detection of substance addiction from primary health care to therapy offices. If you suspect a drug or alcohol problem, there is a simple, easy-to-use screening test—the CAGE questionnaire (see Appendix A)—that can help you assess the presence and extent of a problem. Asking a person the CAGE questionnaire's four questions is an excellent way to screen for alcohol or drug addiction.

The evaluation of potential alcohol and drug problems should be a routine part of an evaluation for all patients who present to a primary care provider or mental health professional. Several studies have shown that the CAGE questionnaire is clinically useful in screening for addiction in a variety of health care settings (Cherpitel, 1999). If a patient has a positive response to two or more questions, then there is an excellent chance that he or she is currently addicted to alcohol or other drugs. A positive response to any one of the four questions raises the issue of alcohol or drug addiction and indicates the need for a full evaluation and an offer of treatment. The key in assessing for addiction in patients who are not presenting for addiction treatment is to maintain a nonjudgmental attitude while obtaining a comprehensive biopsychosocial evaluation. By not focusing exclusively on the alcohol and drug use, one defuses much of the awkwardness of screening for addiction.

Often patients with alcohol or drug problems do not present to health care professionals with initial chief complaints of having an addiction problem. This is especially true for primary care providers and mental health professionals. An important part of the evaluation is to identify symptoms that may indicate a drug problem and be able to ask and obtain necessary information in a nonjudgmental way. Here are two specific examples. This chapter opened with examples of how a patient might initially present to different treatment providers. In the first example, Bill went to his primary care health provider for a routine physical. An opening dialogue could go something like the following:

CLINICIAN: I'm concerned that your liver seems slightly swollen. I'd like to run some tests and ask you a few questions to determine what may be causing it.

BILL: Is it serious?

CLINICIAN: I'm not sure—I won't know until we do some blood work and determine more about what's causing it.

BILL: OK.

CLINICIAN: Drinking can sometimes cause this type of thing. Have you had any alcoholic beverages recently?

BILL: Well, I have a few after work to unwind, but I'm hardly an alcoholic. You know how it is . . . work, the kids, the wife . . .

CLINICIAN: Would you like to know more about where you stand in terms of your drinking—just to be sure it's not endangering your health?

BILL: Well, OK, but I don't have much time. I can't believe my level of drinking is dangerous though.

CLINICIAN: You're probably right. I'd like also to ask a few questions to further assess your drinking. It will only take a minute. Have you ever felt a need to cut down on your drinking?

BILL: I thought I'd cut out drinking for Lent this year but found that after a few days I wasn't feeling quite right, so I went back to my regular amount of drinking.

CLINICIAN: Has anyone annoyed you because he or she complained about your drinking?

BILL: Yes, my wife is on my case all the time. It's getting on my nerves. I'm not an alcoholic; I think she just needs something to complain about.

CLINICIAN: Do you feel guilty about your drinking?

BILL: No, why should I? I don't drink much more than the next guy.

CLINICIAN: Your drinking may or may not be related to your swollen liver. But let's meet again after I get your liver enzyme results, so we know where we stand.

Note how the clinician does not try to force the issue of potential alcohol dependence, but rather stays allied with the patient and simply offers a chance for further information and, most importantly, a return visit.

In the second example that opened this chapter, Alissa initially presents to a mental health professional in a mental health center. With Alissa, the dialogue might proceed the following way:

CLINICIAN: There has been significant weight lost the past several weeks. Is your appetite poor?

ALISSA: No, I'm just eating normally. But sometimes, with the kids running around, I just forget to eat, and you know how that can be. There's so much to do and I'm just chasing them around, and before you know it, it's 10:00 and there's nothing in the house, and I'm exhausted and . . .

CLINICIAN: I'm a bit worried that your weight loss is more than normal and you seem to be somewhat jittery. Are you taking any medications?

ALISSA: Um, well, not really. I mean, I'm not being prescribed anything . . . (looks very anxious).

CLINICIAN: I want to remind you that anything you tell me here is confidential. I'm not going to report it to anyone, but I'm concerned with your rapid weight loss. I'm going to have to ask you some personal questions and I need you to be honest regarding them so that I can treat you, OK?

ALISSA: I can't lose my kids. I just couldn't take it if . . .

CLINICIAN: I promise you that whatever you tell me will not go outside this office without your permission, but if I'm going to help you, I need to know whether or not you are taking drugs of any kind. That's the best way to be sure you will be there for your children. And if you have been taking drugs, it may or may not be related to your other problems.

ALISSA: OK, I smoke crack. Whenever I pick up a pipe, I just can't seem to stop.

CLINICIAN: Most people who use crack find it difficult to stop once a binge begins. Have you been feeling guilty because of your crack use?

ALISSA: Yes, I'm ashamed to tell anyone about it (begins sobbing). My mom was upset when I tried crack a few years ago and I promised her I would never get addicted. Now, crack seems to be the most important thing in the world except for my kids. Even so, I spend all the money I get on crack, and I can't get my kids the right kind of food and clothes because of it. After a binge, I promise myself, that's it . . . but then a few hours later I get cravings, and if I can get a hold of some crack, I'm right back to smoking.

Nonjudgmental Attitude

In order to get an accurate assessment of the patient, your first few steps are crucial in avoiding resistance. In identifying alcohol or drug dependence, it is important to let patients know that you are not going to judge them or release confidential information. This demeanor will encourage patients to trust and confide in you, so that you can have a clear picture of what type of changes will be important over the course of treatment. American society is not empathetic toward people who are addicted to alcohol or drugs. They are typically seen as people who choose to destroy themselves and abandon their families in pursuit of aimless pleasure. Societal attitudes, plus the patient's denial of his or her problems, contribute to patient attempts to hide or minimize alcohol and drug use behaviors. They fear embarrassment, shame, and guilt. Persons using illicit drugs also fear legal consequences in admitting drug use, particularly pregnant women or mothers who could lose custody of their children as a result of disclosure.

CONDUCTING THE COMPREHENSIVE BIOPSYCHOSOCIAL EVALUATION

If the initial screening evaluation suggests an addiction, then you should conduct a comprehensive evaluation that includes consideration of medical, psychological, and social complications. The evaluation of potential alcohol and drug problems is best embedded as part of an evaluation of patients' overall health and well-being. You should emphasize that testing for these problems does not mean that they will be diagnosed with substance addiction. It is simply something either to be "ruled out" or treated, if necessary, as a part of good medical or mental health care.

A comprehensive medical, psychological, and social evaluation is exactly what a **B**iopsychosocial evaluation should involve. Table 3.1 summarizes the key elements of an evaluation. The balance of this chapter discusses the three areas of the evaluation in more detail.

TABLE 3.1. Key Areas of the Biopsychosocial Evaluation

Biological assessment

Questions to ask

General health
>   Have you ever been hospitalized for a medical problem? If so, how many
>   times and what was the nature of the problem?
>   Do you have any chronic medical problems that currently interfere with
>   your life?
>   Are you taking any prescribed medications on a regular basis for a
>   medical problem?
>   Are you currently on medical disability?
>   How often/severe have your medical problems been the past month?

Addiction-related complications
>   Are any medical problems associated with drinking or drug use?
>   Do you have hangovers or feel bad after drinking or drug use?
>   If yes to hangovers, do you experience withdrawal symptoms (e.g., shakes,
>   nausea, gastrointestinal symptoms, seizures, delirium)?

Physical exam (to be conducted by a medical health care provider)

>   Large bruises; evidence of accidents, injuries
>   Tenderness or enlargement of liver
>   Jaundice, abnormal skin tone
>   Small cuts or scarring around major veins (may indicate intravenous drug
>   use)
>   Pupil changes
>   Pinpoint indicates opioid intoxication
>   Dilation indicates stimulant intoxication
>   Obvious behavioral signs of intoxication (e.g., slurred speech,
>   incoordination)
>   Extreme weight loss
>   Nervousness, physical agitation
>   Assess withdrawal symptoms for alcohol

Blood and urine laboratory tests

>   Complete blood count
>   Serum electrolytes and creatinine
>   Lipid profile
>   Liver enzyme tests: GGT, AST (SGOT), ALT (SGPT), bilirubin
>   Hepatitis screening
>   Urine drug screen (after discussing this with the patient)

Psychological assessment

Questions to ask

General mental health
Have you ever been treated for any psychological or emotional problems?
If so, how many times? Are you currently in treatment?
Are you taking any medications for psychological or emotional problems?
During the past month, have you experienced feelings of serious
depression?
During the past month, have you experienced feelings of serious anxiety or
tension?
During the past month, have you experienced trouble understanding,
concentrating, or remembering when you were not using drugs or
drinking alcohol?
During the past month, have you experienced hallucinations or felt
extremely suspicious of others when you were not using drugs or
alcohol?

Psychological distress related to alcohol or drug use
During the past month, have you felt badly about yourself because of
using drugs or drinking?
During the past month, have you lost interest in hobbies or other activities
because of using drugs or drinking?

Mental status exam

Assess for psychiatric emergencies such as suicidal–homicidal ideation.
Assess for psychotic, paranoid symptoms.
Assess for disorientation, delusions.
Assess for symptoms of mood or anxiety disorders.

Administer the Psychological Symptom Inventory—32 (PSI–32)

Administer the Alcohol Use Disorders Identification Test (AUDIT)

Social assessment

Questions to ask

Education/employment
How many years of education have you completed?
Are you currently employed?
If yes, what do you currently do for a living? How many days were you
paid for working? How satisfied are you with your job?
If no, what is your source of economic support? What are your job
prospects?

(*continued on next page*)

TABLE 3.1. (*continued*)

Do you have child-care responsibilities?
If yes, how many children do you care for and what are their ages? Do you
    receive economic support from the father of the child or children?

Marital/relationship status
What is your marital status? How long have you been (single, married,
    separated, divorced)?
Are you satisfied with your marital status?
During the past month, have you had any serious conflicts with your spouse/
    sexual partner?
Whom do you live with? Children (ages)?
Are you satisfied with your current living arrangement?
Do you live with anyone who has a current alcohol or drug problem?
Are there any parenting problems or issues?

Extended family/friends
With whom do you spend most of your free time?
Are you satisfied with spending your free time this way?
Are family/friends supportive of recovery?
Are family/friends aware of addiction problem?
Are family/friends currently drinking excessively or using drugs?
During the past month, have you had any serious conflicts with extended
    family?
During the past month, have you had any serious conflicts with friends or
    coworkers?

Collaboration between Health Care Professionals

It is not expected that every primary care provider, mental health professional, or addiction counselor will feel comfortable with all aspects of the initial comprehensive biopsychosocial evaluation or be able to conduct all aspects of treatment. Ideally, addiction treatment involves a close collaboration between all types of health care professionals. At our treatment research center, we have a team of physicians, nurse practitioners, addiction counselors, social workers, and psychologists who work together to evaluate and provide addiction treatment. A patient typically has one person as his or her primary provider, but other members of the team are integrated into the patient's care as needed. We find that the primary provider can be any member of the team, and the BRENDA approach works well regardless of the background of the primary provider.

Unfortunately, this close collaboration is not always possible, so health care professionals who are not part of an integrated treatment program need to find other health care professionals who can support the BRENDA approach to care. For example, an addiction counselor may establish an addiction treatment program and work closely with physicians in the area to conduct the physical examination, obtain and interpret laboratory tests, and prescribe medication for the patient. Alternatively, primary care providers may include addiction treatment in their practice but work closely with a mental health professional to help evaluate and treat co-occurring mental health problems.

The initial biopsychosocial assessment can be tailored to the type of health care professional who conducts the initial evaluation. As we move through the BRENDA intervention, you will see how to integrate all of these aspects into the recovery plan formulated by you and the patient.

Biological Evaluation

There are no strict rules for the ordering of the biopsychosocial evaluation. In general, however, we find it most helpful to begin by looking at issues of physical health, because many patients who first present for treatment in medical settings are more comfortable seeing their problems as biological. Likewise, for mental health professionals or addiction counselors working with patients who are not specifically presenting for addiction treatment, often, focusing on physical health problems can be easier in starting the assessment. Typically, the biological part of the assessment begins with a thorough history of general, health-related items such as past hospitalizations, chronic problems, use of prescribed medications, and general level of physical functioning (see Table 3.1). Medical problems specifically related to alcohol and other drug use should then be assessed, followed by questions related to the history of the severity of withdrawal symptoms.

Following the history, a medical health care provider should conduct a physical exam, with particular attention to any signs of liver enlargement, jaundice, needle marks or other skin changes, pupil changes, extreme weight loss, and cardiopulmonary abnormalities. Any large bruises or evidence of injuries or accidents (alcohol intoxication is the highest risk factor for industrial accidents) should be noted, as well as any obvious signs of intoxication such as alcohol on the breath or staggering. Jaundice or abnormal skin tone can also indicate an alcohol or drug problem. Pupil dilation should be observed. If pupils are pinpoints and show slowed reaction to light, opiate intoxication is possible. Dilated pupils that show slow reaction to light could be a sign of cocaine or LSD use. Note any abnormal movements or signs of intravenous drug use (small cuts or scarring near major veins). Extreme weight loss may be a sign of stimulant abuse or serious infection such as human immunodeficiency virus (HIV).

Conduct blood tests for liver enzymes (SGOT, GGT, SGPT, uric acid, and bilirubin). Increasingly, a thorough laboratory exam should assess for the presence of hepatitis, particularly hepatitis C. If risk factors are present, HIV testing should also be offered. *Blood or urine screens for drugs and alcohol should not be done without the patient's permission.* If alcohol or drug abuse is suspected, then you may confirm recent drug use with drug screens, but only if the patient agrees. If the patient refuses to have his or her blood or urine tested for alcohol or drugs, then that should be noted but not become a point for debate. Once you have completed the biopsychosocial assessment, you may want to ask the patient for consent to conduct such tests, especially if you think that he or she may not be revealing all relevant information. Typically, once a trusting therapeutic relationship is established, patients will agree to recommended components of treatment, including alcohol and drug testing.

> In the case of Alissa, the mental health professional requested permission for a urine drug screen and also referred her to a collaborating physician for a thorough medical evaluation.

Psychological (Behavioral) Assessment

As part of the biopsychosocial evaluation, the patient needs to be evaluated for symptoms of psychological distress. "Matter-of-factly" ask him or her more questions about drinking and drug use to get a subjective impression and gather information about any substance-related aversive consequences. Frequently, during the physical or psychological evaluation, you can easily interject questions about alcohol and drug use.

Two excellent assessment questionnaires for alcoholism and

other drug use may be used at this point, the CAGE, mentioned earlier, and the Alcohol Use Disorders Identification Test (AUDIT; see Appendix A). If the patient seems afraid of an addiction diagnosis, you should probably start with the AUDIT, which is more quantitative and less likely to scare the patient into lying to protect him- or herself. Both questionnaires are brief and easy to administer. By beginning the psychological assessment with these questionnaires, which largely deal with frequency, amount, and reasons for drinking, you can quickly determine a great deal about the problem. Both of these screens are designed just for alcohol problems, but you can use modified versions to test for other substances if you suspect they may be involved.

After an assessment of alcohol and drug use, it is important to determine if the patient is suffering from any psychiatric symptoms. Depression and anxiety are the most common psychiatric symptoms that occur in conjunction with substance dependence. Less frequent, but still common, is paranoia. Sometimes these symptoms disappear with abstinence, but if symptoms persist and go untreated, or if there is a pervasive underlying psychiatric disorder, such conditions will almost certainly provoke a relapse to drinking or drug use.

Patients may be anxious about being screened for mental illness and believe that just because you want to test them, it means that you think they are "crazy." Reassure them that this is not the case, and that though some of the questions may seem unusual, it is important to have the fullest picture of the patient to facilitate their getting needed treatment. To assess the extent and type of psychological symptoms, use the Psychological Symptom Inventory—32 (PSI-32; see Appendix A). In some cases, a formal psychiatric interview may be indicated, and a psychiatrically trained professional should be asked to determine if there is an underlying psychiatric disorder. If you find some serious psychiatric problems beyond substance dependence that you have not been trained to treat, you should make every attempt to refer patients for the needed treatment while they continue to see you for treatment of their substance dependence.

In addition to biological and psychological issues, assessment should also look at social factors. Does the patient have a job? What kind of family and/or social support does the patient have available? Will social factors aid or impede his or her recovery?

Social Assessment

Social factors play key roles in a patient's treatment success or failure. One of the best predictors of long-term recovery is whether or not the patient has a job (Carver & Dunham, 1991). Unemployment may have resulted from uncontrollable drinking or drug use and can be a direct signal of the severity of the dependence. Also, if the patient is unemployed, there is more free time to pursue obtaining and consuming substances. Sometimes a consistent history of unemployment can be a cause of underlying substance dependence and increase the risk for relapse. In many cases, people without jobs form their identities based on a career of drugs and alcohol. Recovery may not be possible if these social factors are not addressed, so learning about them early in treatment and helping the patient realize their relationship with the substance problem are important.

Although you probably will not get a full social assessment in your first interview, you most definitely should ask about employment status, the nature of the patient's work, job satisfaction, and stresses. It is also important to try to determine how the patient sees his or her future; for example, does it include a career?

Another consideration is the patient's family and marital status. Are there marital stresses and does the spouse drink or use drugs? Are there children, and if so, how is the patient functioning as a parent? For younger patients, parental relationships may be a causal factor in why they drink or use, so this must also be considered.

The patient's larger social milieu should also be noted. Where does the patient drink or take drugs and with whom? How important a role do drinking and drug taking play in his or her social life? Again, quitting is more difficult if patients have to abandon their entire social circle. Thus, it is important to get a sense of which factors may be most important in each individual case.

Do take note of any remarks made by the patient that offer insight into job or social situations, and follow the patient's lead as to what he or she is willing to discuss. If he or she is defensive or unwilling to discuss certain topics, leave them for later visits.

When all elements of the biopsychosocial evaluation are complete and the results obtained, the clinician needs to consider their significance and then report the findings to the patient. The next chapter describes the preparation and presentation of the report.

CHAPTER 4

The Report

How to Prepare and Present the Assessment Results

Upon physical examination, Bill winces during your palpation of his abdomen, though he denies pain when you ask if it is tender. You also observe a slight swelling in the area that is most tender to your touch. Bill's liver enzymes are seriously elevated and he has three positive items on the CAGE assessment, including difficulty cutting down on his drinking, feeling annoyed by his wife's criticism, and using alcohol to reduce withdrawal symptoms. He is drinking six to ten drinks per day but denies problems with work and does not show significant symptoms of psychological distress. His PSI score is only a 6. However, his wife has expressed concern about his drinking and this has led to frequent arguments.

Alissa's urine screen is positive for cocaine. She reports that she has been smoking crack cocaine on weekends and frequently spends almost her entire welfare check on purchasing cocaine, leaving her low on money for food and other necessities. She says her boyfriend smokes cocaine as well. Her medical evaluation reveals a yeast infection that has not responded to treatment. When the health care provider asked if she would agree to an HIV test, she refused. Her liver enzymes are elevated and she reports using alcohol "to come down off the pipe."

Stephen was initially evaluated by the company nurse before referral to the EAP. The nurse's evaluation shows that Stephen's liver enzymes are slightly above normal but not significantly elevated. However, the BAC (blood-alcohol concentration) test run by the nurse after his accident was positive for alcohol. He also has mentioned to the EAP counselor that his boss has "been on his case" about lateness and absenteeism.

The **R**eport stage in BRENDA involves more than simply reporting the assessment findings to the patient. Rather, there are three important steps: (1) formulating a patient profile from the assessment results, (2) presenting the results of the assessment in such a way that the patient can understand the results, and (3) observing the patient's reaction to the report with respect to motivation to change his or her behavior. While many patients suspect they have problems with alcohol or drug use, often hearing someone express this problem can elicit a strong negative reaction that can take the form of anger, denial, anxiety, depression, guilt, or any combination of these feelings. In contrast to other programs that put the full responsibility to cope with these feelings on the patient, the BRENDA model helps patients cope with these feelings. Often a patient's way of coping with this emotional distress is to run away and avoid these feelings (denial). The treatment provider using the BRENDA model attempts to minimize the strong negative reaction in the **R**eport stage and to help the patient cope with the emotional distress but not avoid it in the **E**mpathy stage. Let us turn our attention to preparing and presenting the results of the biopsychosocial assessment.

FORMULATING A PROFILE

Is There an Alcohol or Drug Problem?

Once the assessment has been completed, a full picture of the patient should begin to emerge. As you formulate a profile on your patient, the first question to ask yourself is whether the person is addicted to a substance. As we discussed earlier, addiction involves three criteria: (1) impaired control, (2) biopsychosocial consequences, and (3) an addictive cycle in which drug use creates a need for more drug use. In each of the three cases that begin this chapter, we see that the patients have symptoms from each criterion. Bill has unsuccessfully tried to stop drinking for periods of time; his drinking has led to medical problems and contributes to problems in his relationship with his wife. He stated that he returned to drinking to reduce feelings of distress after a brief period of abstinence. All of these symptoms point to a diagnosis of alcohol addiction. Alissa presents a clear picture of cocaine addiction. She cannot control her use of crack once a binge starts. Her cocaine use has had severe social consequences in terms of caring for her children and may even lead her to lose custody of them. Alissa uses crack to reduce the craving and is clearly stuck in an addictive cycle in which crack use leads to more crack use. Stephen's situation is not so clearly defined. His alcohol use is associated with an accident at work and his boss is clearly upset with his drinking. So while he has one of the three criteria for addiction, it is not clear whether he can control his drinking or use alcohol to reduce craving or withdrawal symptoms.

Severity of Biopsychosocial Complications

The diagnosis of alcohol and drug dependence is merely the first step in formulating a report. If we compare the situations of Bill and Alissa, for example, we see a very different picture. Bill's addiction to alcohol may be as severe as Alissa's addiction to crack, but his overall emotional, social, occupational, and physical health is much better than hers. At our center we assess the relative severity of problems for an individual along seven dimensions: (1) alcohol problems, (2) drug problems, (3) employment problems, (4) physical health problems, (5) emotional distress, (6) social interactions, and (7) legal problems. Bill has moderate problems in the alcohol, medical, and social areas but is currently relatively free of problems in other areas. In contrast, Alissa has problems across the entire range, including the beginning of an alcohol problem; she is financially and emotionally distressed, with few job prospects and social support; her physical health may be compromised by HIV infection, and she faces legal difficulties with respect to keeping custody of her children.

The comprehensive biopsychosocial evaluation thus leads to very different profiles for each patient seeking treatment. In BRENDA, the wide variability in the clinical presentation for each patient means that the approach to treatment will differ accordingly. Yet for many treatment programs, once a diagnosis of dependence is made, the treatment recommendation is the same: Stop using alcohol and other drugs, and go to community meetings of support groups. We review the treatment options in a subsequent chapter, but for now, it is enough to note that different addiction profiles create the need for different treatment approaches.

REPORTING THE RESULTS

Once you have assessed your patients and have had a chance to formulate a profile, you will Report the results to them and discuss the implications of the results. Again, it is extremely important to remain nonjudgmental and matter-of-fact. For most patients, hearing that they have a drinking or drug problem can be emotionally upsetting. The more you convey your comfort with treating this problem within the context of good health practices, the more likely they will be open to hearing what you have to say and accepting your help. Also, by listening to a patient's reactions upon hearing his or her Report, you can acquire a greater understanding of his or her motivation to change the behavior and the individual Needs for wanting to change. Observing the reaction to the biopsychosocial report is important in determining what will best help the patient recover. While the health care provider may be doing most of the talking, it is the reaction to the Report that guides the subsequent components of treatment. The following examples illustrate that providing feedback to a patient is an interactive process.

Here is how the dialogue with Bill might begin:

CLINICIAN: I have your test results. Your liver enzyme levels are significantly higher than normal. Based on how you described your pattern of alcohol use, I believe your drinking is the most likely cause.

BILL: That can't be. I am not some Bowery bum alcoholic. I mean, I don't drink more than any of my friends . . . I have a good job . . . there must be some mistake.

CLINICIAN: I agree with you. You are not some Bowery alcoholic. You are a successful businessman who has had trouble controlling your drinking on occasion, whose drinking is of concern to your wife, and who has liver damage most likely related to drinking. On the other hand, drinking has not affected your work and except for your liver, you appear to be in good physical health.

BILL: (*responds to the clinician's* **R***eport with continuing skepticism, but finally asks:*) Well, what are my options here?

Notice that rather than argue with Bill, the clinician agrees with Bill's observation that he does not fit the description of an alcoholic and matter-of-factly restates the highlights of the biopsychosocial evaluation. We can summarize the important components of presenting the **R**eport to the patient:

1. Your initial report should stick to reporting the facts that support the existence of an alcohol or drug problem. Do not argue with the patient; rather, just keep reiterating that the problem is real.
2. Do not make judgments about the problem or immediately offer any specific advice on what to do about it.
3. Give the patient time to react and be open to his or her emotional response.

OBSERVING THE PATIENT'S REACTION TO THE REPORT (ASSESSING STAGE OF CHANGE)

Attending to the patient's reaction to your **R**eport is an important part of the BRENDA model. It will tell you a great deal about what degree of resistance he or she has toward getting help. By understanding the patient's perspective, you can more easily overcome resistance to change. In the past, some addiction counselors might have recommended further confrontation, trying to make Bill accept rather than "deny" that he has a problem with alcohol. But research has shown that acceptance of the label "alcoholic" is not essential to recovery (Miller, 1995). The patient will be more motivated to accept what you are saying if you do not spend time arguing about whether or not he or she is an "alcoholic"; rather, clearly and straightforwardly present the results of the evaluation.

Preparing to Change

Bill's reaction to the report initially caused some discomfort and resistance, but with nonjudgmental persistence on the part of the clinician, Bill was able to see that he had a problem and ask for help. According to the stages of change assessment, we would say that Bill was in the "preparation" stage. This is an example of how the presentation of the **R**eport prepared the patient actively to change his or her behavior. However, it does not always happen so easily.

Contemplation: Ambivalent about Change

In the following example of dialogue, a crucial part of the **R**eport is presented to Alissa, who is in the stage of "contemplation" but needs to move into the "preparation" stage before she can change her behavior:

CLINICIAN: I'd like to review with you your urine test results.

ALISSA: I know, I know, positive for cocaine, right? What am I going to do? I have to stop, I know, but how? My boyfriend sells it, and when it's in the house, I don't know how to say no. I've tried before but I always seem to go back to it. I did think about leaving him, and almost did once . . . but he pays for food and so much stuff for the kids, I just can't do without him either! I'd like to stop smoking crack but I just can't see myself stopping now.

Alissa knows she has a problem and wants to change but is skeptical about her ability to do so. To move into the stage of "preparation," she first needs to feel supported in her choice to get well. She will also need to learn that she has alternatives and that she is capable of pursuing them successfully.

Contemplators tend to have at least thought about the possibility that they might have a problem. However, they have not yet decided whether they will accept the idea or do anything to change their behavior. They are typically ambivalent (i.e., unsure if the evidence necessitates change) and also afraid that if they try to change and fail, it will be too great a blow to their self-esteem. To motivate contemplators, try to help them understand that change is necessary, and that they are capable of changing. For comtemplators, a sort of cost–benefit analysis is taking place. The **R**eport just presented can give weight to the costs of addiction but to tip the scales in favor of taking action, special attention should be given to an understanding of the patient's own reasons for treating the addiction: the Needs assessment. In Chapter 4, we look at how best to provide Alissa with the support and encouragement she needs to decide to change her drug use and related behaviors. In Chapters 5 and 6, we explore Alissa's specific needs and her options for best meeting those needs.

Finally, there are patients like Stephen, who, even after being presented with the results of the biopsychosocial assessment, are not convinced that the results show a problem with alcohol or drug use.

Precontemplation: Adamant against Change

Stephen is a precontemplator as his response to his Report shows.

CLINICIAN: Well, I've got your Report, Stephen. While there are no laboratory or physical problems associated with excessive drinking, you tell me that you have had three alcohol-related accidents in the last 2 years. From what you have told me about your drinking, I see that you binge several times a month and during these binges, you have driven while intoxicated and have had these couple of accidents. This suggests to me that you may have a drinking problem.

STEPHEN: I don't want to stop drinking. It's how I socialize . . . it is how I relax. Thanks for the advice, but I really don't want to quit.

CLINICIAN: I understand that you find alcohol drinking enjoyable. However, your binges have led to several accidents and Monday-morning hangovers at work. If you continue to binge drink, you may lose your job.

STEPHEN: I don't care about my job. I'd rather quit my job than give up drinking.

Stephen is firmly planted in the precontemplation stage, though it appears that he at one time thought about stopping. For patients in the precontemplation stage, many treatment programs would simply drop the issue and tell patients to come back when they were ready for treatment. The BRENDA model, however, sees this stage as a fairly common challenge to the clinician and proceeds to help move the patient along to the next stage of treatment. Even with a direct and nonjudgmental approach to presenting his report, Stephen is not ready to accept that he has an alcohol problem. To push the issue further at this time would likely lead to anger and a lost opportunity to engage Stephen in treatment. In the next chapter, we will see how Empathy and a Needs assessment help the clinician find a way to move Stephen from the precontemplation to the contemplation stage and to forge a therapeutic relationship to keep Stephen in treatment. Over time, Stephen can move from the contemplation to preparation and action stages as the clinician continues to use the BRENDA method.

As we shall see within each individual session, all stages of BRENDA are at least touched upon; however, in the early stages of treatment, the Biopsychosocial assessment and the Report stages are especially important, particularly for patients who deny they have a disorder, or who, after a period of abstinence, relapse and want to discontinue medication and treatment sessions. But even for patients who are doing well in treatment, the Report can provide feedback that the interventions are having a positive impact. This feedback can give people a sense of accomplishment and motivate further changes.

TABLE 4.1. How to Determine Which "Stage of Change" a Person Is In

1. Did the person solve the problem more than 6 months ago? Yes No
2. Did the person take action on the problem in the past 6 months? Yes No
3. Does the person intend to take action now? Yes No
4. Does the person recognize a problem but is not ready to take action? Yes No

"No" to all questions:	Precontemplation
"No" to all except question 4:	Contemplation
"No" to only questions 1 and 2:	Determination/preparation
"Yes" to question 2, "No" to question 1:	Action
"Yes" to question 1:	Maintenance

Note. Based on Prochaska (1994).

CHAPTER 5

Empathetic Understanding

Listening to the Patient

Bill is concerned about his elevated liver enzymes but is also feeling shame about his inability to control his drinking. He is fearful that being in treatment will interfere with his job and lead to more social shame and stigma. Ultimately, he is concerned that alcohol drinking or engaging in treatment will lead to loss of the lifestyle he has obtained.

Alissa reveals more about her relationship with her boyfriend, the crack cocaine dealer. He has hit her several times and has at least one other girlfriend. She feels trapped in the relationship. Tearfully, she expresses feelings of helplessness and despair.

Stephen remains adamant that he will not give up alcohol. When the therapist points out that his drinking may cost him his job, he expresses anger, keeps glancing at his watch, and seems anxious to leave.

EMPATHETIC LISTENING STRATEGIES

Empathetic understanding will help you connect with patients in every aspect of the BRENDA cycle, but it is particularly critical at the juncture where you are listening and responding to patients' reactions to their **R**eports. When people have been told that they have a substance dependence problem, and they begin to realize the potential consequences this could have, they usually becomes extremely uncomfortable. This discomfort can make or break the early stages of treatment. It is usually experienced when someone is moving from contemplation to preparation. In order to help patients, you need to let them know that you understand what they are going through and why they feel the way they do. Research has found that substance dependence counselors who get the best results are those who are most empathetic toward their patients—that is, those who listen, show understanding of the patient's problems, and are supportive (Miller, Benefield, et al., 1993).

Collaboration versus Confrontation

If you try to impose advice without empathy, and simply tell patients what to do, then you will provoke resistance. Empathetic practitioners avoid power struggles by allying themselves with their patients and recognizing that the more understood people feel, the more likely they will be to listen to advice with an open mind and follow it.

First, allow enough time in the visit for the patient to express him- or herself and react to the **R**eport. As you present your **R**eport, listen carefully to the patient's reactions and concerns. To maximize empathy, you also need to get a sense of what is most and least important to the patient. This will be the basis for the next BRENDA stage, which is looking at patient **N**eeds, and reframing these needs in a way that will allow change to happen. Sometimes the **E**mpathic stage of BRENDA will require literally minutes, and, in other cases, several visits. This is because some patients may need constant reminders of the results in the **R**eport (due to strong denial), which, in turn, can require your continual reassurances and support in order for them to want to change their behavior.

Fear Reduction: Coping or Avoidance?

Miller has observed that there are two ways people can reduce the discomfort of the realization that they have a problem. They can either reduce their risky behaviors (stop taking drugs or cut down drinking amounts) or reduce the fear they relate to it (Miller, 1995). People try to reduce their fear with denial, minimization, rationalization, and avoidance of help. They react this way when the fear is too great and when they have no other coping resources or emotional support. However, if patients feel that their problems are understood and there is no reason to feel ashamed about talking about the problem, you will not observe much denial, minimization, or rationalization.

Building Up versus Breaking Down

Patients also need to feel that they are capable of change, and that life without drugs and alcohol will be bearable. They look to you for these feelings. Your optimism about their recovery will go a long way toward helping them incorporate this feeling and own it. Therefore, through Empathetic understanding, you can help support the belief that they have the ability to recover. Often, by being presented a series of small steps toward recovery, patients can begin to visualize that recovery is possible. By getting a sense of their Needs, you can help ensure that the treatment helps them reach their life goals.

APPLYING EMPATHY

A Report that gives evidence of an alcohol or drug problem will arouse anxiety in the patient. This anxiety can provide a motivation to deal with the problem and is the best-case scenario. The patient may, however, deal with the anxiety by denying or avoiding the problem. Empathy helps the patient cope with the anxiety and lessens the tendency to avoid.

Coping with Anxiety

In Bill's case, it is worth exploring what is causing his anxiety as the therapist presents the Report to him. An Empathetic understanding of his situation reveals that he is willing to explore a change in his drinking habits but may not be willing to call himself an "alcoholic."

CLINICIAN: How are you feeling right now?

BILL: I guess I'm a little stunned and frightened. As you point out, I may have a problem with alcohol. I guess I sort of suspected as much but I didn't want to think about it. What will people think? I'm the CEO of a big company. What if I have to go away for a month, and everyone will know I'm an alcoholic? I could lose my job, my income, my lifestyle. Oh, God, what's wrong with me?

It is clear from this exchange that Bill fears threatening his entire lifestyle by acknowledging he has a problem drinking. In his mind, he immediately goes from a drinking problem to becoming a severe alcoholic living on the streets. Rather than contemplate his problem, he has tried to minimize and deny it. At this point, the clinician can first empathize with him by stating that given his assumptions, one can understand why he would be fearful. Also it is helpful to explore any other feeling or reasons for distressing feelings.

CLINICIAN: I can understand why you are feeling anxious, if you see anyone with a drinking problem as heading down a road of living in the Bowery, and then you fear loss of the wonderful lifestyle you are currently living. Is there anything else about having a drinking problem that bothers you?

BILL: Yes, I feel ashamed. I should be able to control my drinking on my own. Yet here I am, talking with my doctor about this. I make important decisions all day. I run a successful company. Why can't I simply decide to stop drinking so much? Why can't I control my drinking?

CLINICIAN: You are a very successful businessman and can control many things in your life. I can understand why you are feeling confused and ashamed about not being able to control your drinking when there are so many other areas of your life that you can control.

Challenging Fear-Eliciting Assumptions

After giving patients an opportunity to express their feelings, the clinician should encourage effective coping by challenging the assumptions that lead to the distressing feelings. Often, patients assume that people with alcohol or other drug problems are morally bad, weak-willed, hopeless, or fundamentally flawed. By presenting a model that does not blame patients for their addiction, and by offering hope, one can effectively change these assumptions and reduce distressing feelings such as fear, guilt, and shame. For example, the clinician's response to Bill might be the following:

CLINICIAN: I have treated many successful businessmen who, like yourself, had alcohol problems. Often, they felt fearful that people would look at them differently once aware that they had a drinking problem. Some were fearful that their drinking would inevitably lead to a loss of their job and family. All were confused as to why they could not control their drinking when they had such excellent control in other areas of their lives. It surprised them to find that they could deal with their problem without it progressing and that the people around them with whom they shared their problem were very supportive.

BILL: But why can't I control my drinking when so many others can?

CLINICIAN: It's not certain why some people find it difficult to control their drinking while others do not, but our scientific understanding of addiction suggests that it is not your fault. Rather, your body probably responds to alcohol differently than other people's, and it makes it more difficult for you to stop drinking once you begin a binge. Also, your body has learned that when you feel a little shaky the next day, you can take away these withdrawal symptoms by drinking. Therefore, when you are feeling a little shaky, it is the most natural thing to drink to take the shakes away.

BILL: I'm feeling a bit better. Maybe I can do something about this problem before it gets worse.

CLINICIAN: Bill, I am confident that you will successfully deal with this problem just as you have dealt with the problems you have faced in business. We will work on this together.

From Ambivalence to Preparation

Alissa is ambivalent about changing her behavior. While she sees that she has a problem, a serious problem at that, she sees no way to get out of her situation. She is quite despondent, and a life without crack and alcohol seems impossible. For Alissa, the **E**mpathy stage is critical to help her prepare to begin treatment. Particularly important is to build up her hope and confidence.

CLINICIAN: You look tearful. What's bothering you?

ALISSA: I just don't see much hope. My life is a mess and now I stand to lose my children. I just want to escape.

CLINICIAN: I can see why you may feel trapped, since you live with an abusive boyfriend and have limited resources in order to get away from the situation. Maybe there are resources that we can use to help turn things around. Is there any close friend or relative that you can call on to help? Maybe even move in with temporarily?

ALISSA: Well, my aunt will be disappointed to learn that I'm using crack again, but she once said that she would put me up if I needed a place to stay.

CLINICIAN: Yes, your aunt sounds like a wonderful resource. Are there other supports that you can call on now?

ALISSA: Well I have a friend who is recovering and she is drug-free. She went to a church that helped her get clean. I guess it's possible to get better, but I'm just not sure it's worth it. After a couple of hits on the crack pipe, I feel so good.

Alissa has begun to feel a sense of hope, but her ambivalence about giving up crack is apparent.

CLINICIAN: Yes, of course, it's possible to get better. But it is also possible to stay where you are. Smoking crack does give you some relief, but only for a brief period of time. What are some of the reasons you want to stop smoking crack?

ALISSA: I mostly feel miserable now and I want to get better. It's no solution. I want to be there for my kids. I want to feel proud about my life. I have tried to stop smoking so often. I'm afraid I'll fail again. I just can't deal with another failure.

CLINICIAN: I know you have not been able to give up crack on your own, and I can understand your fear of having another failure. There are no guarantees, Alissa, but know that you have supports in your life. Your aunt and friend sound like they could be a big help. Also, I am here to help you. Together we'll find a way out of this situation.

ALISSA: (*Smiles through tears*) Thank you.

Collaboration

For some individuals, a presentation of the results of the assessment does not lead to a motivated patient, but rather may lead to a further resolution to deny that a problem exists. Stephen is a good example of such a patient. In many treatment approaches, one would try to argue with him until he realized that the consequences of his drinking were severe enough to warrant quitting. But the BRENDA model assumes that the clinician can and should facilitate the patient's motivation to obtain treatment. An important approach is to collaborate with patients in an Empathetic understanding of their problems from their own perspective. So, for example, a man who is adamant about completely giving up alcohol can be offered a program that will help him try to reduce drinking and the negative consequences of alcohol in his life, without requiring him to give up alcohol entirely. If he fails at a moderate drinking program, he is much more likely to accept that he must abstain and work toward a goal of abstinence.

Let us look at what an empathetic response to Stephen might be like.

CLINICIAN: How do you feel about what this Report says?

STEPHEN: Well, on paper, that guy looks like an alcoholic and I don't like it. I don't want to stop drinking. I don't want to be sitting around church basements for the rest of my life saying, "I'm Stephen and I'm an alcoholic." I'm too young to be that dull.

CLINICIAN: It sounds like you are not interested in going to AA meetings. I can understand that not everyone fits into this type of approach to treatment. What if there were a program to help you reduce your drinking just enough to solve your problems at work? Would you consider trying that?

STEPHEN: You mean without quitting drinking?

CLINICIAN: Yes, the program would help you cut down on the amount you drink.

STEPHEN: And that's it?

CLINICIAN: That would be up to you. You could decide what the ultimate goal would be.

STEPHEN: Well, that sounds too easy!

CLINICIAN: No program to reduce drinking is easy. However, since your blood-alcohol level was so high in your accident report, I suspect your boss might recommend some sort of program before you can return to work. This type of program might be a good choice for you.

STEPHEN: And that type of program would count?

CLINICIAN: If you did not test positive for alcohol at work again. You would be making important changes.

STEPHEN: I could do that, I guess. I mean, I really don't want to keep messing up, do I?

CLINICIAN: No, and I think you are a very good candidate for this program.

As you can see, the clinician takes his or her lead from Stephen and suggests an approach that is most likely to appeal to his needs. The clinician is realistic and encouraging, not trying to force Stephen into doing anything he does not want. BRENDA practitioners do not act as agents for anyone but the patients themselves. Their first mission is to state clearly and straightforwardly to the patient how they see the problem.

The clinician reframes the patient's concerns and reinforces the idea that he or she can get better. When there is resistance, the clinician does not argue but simply moves on to another area. Because patients expect to be forced into one particular way of dealing with a drug or alcohol problem, they are surprised, and much more willing, when offered options that are congruent with their own goals. This is what true Empathetic understanding fosters.

In summary, Empathetic understanding helps reduce the patient's discomfort, builds collaboration, and increases optimism that recovery is possible. Together, patient and clinician create a strong therapeutic alliance that prevents denial and avoidance of the problem. In the next chapter, we discuss how the Needs can be made more explicit and lead to direct advice regarding treatment options.

CHAPTER 6

▆▆▆

Needs

Identifying Patient Needs and Priorities

While initially adamant that he is not an alcoholic, Bill believes he may have a drinking problem. He is concerned about his pattern of daily drinking and the irritable feeling he experiences if he goes a day without drinking. He is determined to find a way to do something about his drinking before it leads to more significant problems, yet he does not want others to know about his drinking problem.

Alissa feels overwhelmed. While she stopped crying and has listened to reassurances that she can get better, Alissa is afraid that nothing will be able to help her. Also, several of her friends have made repeated attempts at treatment without success.

Stephen has doubts that he needs help in controlling his drinking because he sees his accidents as rare occurrences. But because he knows he will have to show that he is getting some kind of help in order to keep his job, he is willing to continue seeing the clinician.

Identifying and prioritizing each of these patients' Needs are the keys to helping them accept treatment. A need exists when there is impairment in the overall health or the development and growth of the individual seeking treatment. Now that you have access to the results of the patient's **B**iopsychosocial evaluation and his or her response to the **Re**port, you should be able to get a sense of which **N**eeds have more priority for the patient than others. We discuss two basic kinds of **N**eeds that patients present for treatment. Basic health safety needs refer to the current medical and psychosocial health of the patient. Patient needs reflect the hopes and desires of the patient.

IDENTIFYING NEEDS

The identification of **N**eeds is an ongoing process that begins with the biopsychosocial evaluation but continues throughout the **R**eporting of the evaluation and the **E**mpathetic understanding of the patient's response to the report. Many of the health safety needs are apparent during the physical examination and the psychosocial evaluation. Other **N**eeds will emerge over the course of using the BRENDA method. There are also "rare" times when the clinician must unilaterally decide what course of action is necessary, for example, when there is imminent threat to the life of the patient. However, the general philosophy of the BRENDA model is that the **N**eeds reflect collaboration between the clinician and patient. The following general list gives an overview of the health safety needs (medical and psychosocial) a clinician looks for:

Medical management of alcohol or other drug withdrawal symptoms

Medical management of physical conditions caused by acute or chronic alcohol or drug use

Psychiatric management of serious mental disorders

Learning appropriate coping skills to deal with psychological stress arising from employment or family/relationship issues

A safe social environment in which recovery can take place

Alternative sources of pleasurable activities to replace alcohol or drug use

Hope and confidence to obtain needs and recover successfully

Let us now turn our attention to some specific types of **N**eeds that the patient may present and ways to elicit underlying needs that may not be obvious from the initial presentation.

BASIC HEALTH AND SAFETY NEEDS

Medical Emergencies

The first priority must be the health and safety of the patient. If, for example, Bill came to his appointment complaining of vomiting blood, and appeared pale and lightheaded, the clinician must rule out a serious medical emergency such as internal bleeding. For health care professionals who do not have medical training, it is important to have an available colleague to consult for medical emergencies. One important advantage of working with a team of health care providers is that the medical assessment and treatment can be seamlessly integrated among psychologists, social workers, and addiction counselors. You may encounter medical emergencies rarely in your practice, but the security of having a medical backup will help relieve your concerns and fears, and those of your patient. It is beyond the scope of this manual to review all the medical emergencies, including managing severe withdrawal that can accompany chronic alcohol and drug abuse. It is important, however, to ensure the physical health of the patient.

Psychosocial Crises

Many patients first present for treatment during some psychosocial crisis in their lives. For example, Alissa may be concerned for her own welfare because her boyfriend has threatened to kill her if she decides to leave him. Just as it is helpful to have medical backup for nonmedically trained providers, it is also helpful to have social workers, psychologists, and/or psychiatrists who can be called upon for crisis intervention. Another factor that demands immediate attention is the threat of suicide or homicide. About half of all completed suicides and murders are associated with alcohol or drug intoxication. If Alissa feel helpless and hopeless about her situation, she may see suicide as her only way out. It is beyond the scope of this manual to review all psychiatric conditions or emergencies that can accompany chronic alcohol and drug abuse. It is important, however, to be able to recognize an emergency and know when immediate referral or hospitalization may be necessary.

PATIENT NEEDS AND PRIORITIES

While medical and psychosocial emergencies may demand immediate attention and dictate the early needs of the patient, patients often present without any obvious and immediate reason to give up their drug use. Also, when the immediate threat to survival is gone, some patients may lose their motivation to continue treatment. For this reason, a strategy to enlist the collaboration of patients in identifying their needs can facilitate treatment retention. Finding this hook for treatment must be approached from the patient's perspective. While the biopsychosocial assessment may reveal problems in several areas, only those areas that are identified by the patient as important will be crucial in motivating treatment compliance. Other treatment programs talk about the need for the patient to hit "rock bottom" as a prerequisite to begin treatment. Often, "rock bottom" occurs only after there are casualties in relationships, lost job opportunities, or even medical complications including death. The BRENDA approach assumes that a skillful approach to treatment can help motivate patients to change their behavior before experiencing such severe complications. By obtaining a thorough **B**iopsychosocial assessment, reporting that information in a nonjudgmental way to the patient, and understanding the symptoms from the patient's perspective to identify his or her primary needs, one can enlist the cooperation of the patient.

As you begin to understand the problem from the biopsychosocial assessment and the patient's perspective; the needs for each individual become increasingly clear. Needs are further discussed and agreed upon in the **N**eeds assessment. It is at the synthesis of the **B**iopsychosocial assessment and **E**mpathy stage, that a broad outline of **N**eeds is uncovered.

Let's look now at determining the patient **N**eeds of each of our three patient examples.

Bill

For example, Bill's **B**iopsychosocial assessment reveals a history of daily drinking, with use of alcohol to avoid possible withdrawal symptoms. The physical exam shows evidence of mild withdrawal including a slight tremor, rapid heart rate, and sweating. The exam and laboratory tests also reveal evidence of alcohol liver disease. From the clinician's perspective, the acute problem of alcohol withdrawal is a possible safety issue and must be addressed. The liver damage is less critical to address immediately and is likely to improve as Bill reduces or abstains from alcohol. The Report and Empathy stages show that Bill is fearful of losing his lifestyle and feels embarrassment over not being able to control his drinking. While a medical practitioner may be more concerned about the elevated liver enzymes results, for Bill, that may not be the hook to engage him in treatment. Bill seems determined and motivated to engage in treatment, especially if his fears and concerns are addressed.

Health safety needs

- Alcohol detoxification
- Probable alcohol induced liver disease

Patient needs

- Does not wish to be considered an alcoholic
- Not totally opposed to abstinence
- May be interested in improving his relationship with his wife

Alissa

For Alissa, the issues are different. It would be desirable for her to have some distance from her boyfriend so she can experience some extended abstinence and also have the opportunity to look at things from a more objective viewpoint. At the same time, it is clear that her children are her most important concern because she is afraid that her drug use may cause her to lose custody of them. Inpatient rehabilitation may be ideal, provided child-care arrangements can be arranged while she is in the hospital. She also is likely to go along with this suggestion given that she believes that if she keeps using cocaine, she may lose her children. Looking at it from her point of view, family and social concerns—the kids, the boyfriend, the fact that she is unemployed and has little education—are going to be crucial in determining her course of recovery. Thus, if you offer her treatment that does not take her relationship with her children into consideration, she is likely to think that nobody really understands her situation. In fact, you are likely to lose her as a patient and could push her motivation from the determination back to the contemplation stage of change.

Health safety needs

- Needs a change in environment due to live-in drug dealer boyfriend
- May need antidepressant treatment for depression

Patient needs

- Primary concern is her children
- Requires child care to attend inpatient treatment
- Needs extra support to see that treatment can work
- May need job training/help returning to school

Stephen

Stephen may be willing to reduce the frequency and the consequences of binges, but he is also clear on not wanting to stop drinking completely. One can debate the relative merits of a program where reduced drinking is the goal. However, if Stephen drops out of treatment, then it is unlikely his drinking problems will improve, especially considering his previous failed attempts to cut down on his own. For some people, the best we can do in the early stages of treatment is to move someone from precontemplation to contemplation. At least Stephen is willing to take some steps to reduce his drinking in the context of a treatment plan.

Health safety needs

- Reduce episodes of bingeing that are associated with industrial accidents

Patient needs

- Primary concern is that he will be asked to give up drinking
- Concerned that he will be labeled an alcoholic and lose his job
- Learning to enjoy life without bingeing on alcohol
- Needs support for a drinking-in-moderation program

Remember that it is what the patient considers important, not what you consider important that counts. Looking at Stephen's situation from the outside, for example, you might think that giving up drinking entirely is the more sensible course to take. But that is your judgment, not his, and if you try to impose this upon him, you have no chance of reaching him.

The same is true for Alissa and Bill. Both have Needs that are not obvious unless you listen closely to their own descriptions of their situations and concerns.

To develop a proper treatment plan for your patients, you also have to know what treatment options are available and which are most useful in meeting a patient's specific Needs. These are listed and briefly described in the next chapter on Direct advice.

CHAPTER 7

Direct Advice

Matching Needs to Treatment Options

Now that you have a good picture of your patients' **N**eeds and their stage of change (or level of motivation), you can offer **D**irect advice to guide them in their recovery. Research finds that patients given a menu of treatment options have improved treatment retention and treatment outcomes compared to patients who are simply told what to do (Larimer & Marlatt, 1990). Keep this in mind as you consider what you will offer each patient. Remember that the more options you provide, the better sense patients will have that they are choosing their own goals and methods of change. This will allow them to be more committed to treatment and the process they need to go through in order to change.

The best way to determine which options are most suitable is to familiarize the patient with the available resources. In this chapter, we give an overview of the treatment options. You can obtain more information from the National Institute on Alcohol Abuse and Alcoholism (NIAAA), and the National Institute on Drug Abuse (NIDA) (see also Volpicelli & Szalavitz, 2000).

Consideration of the best treatment options should ideally be based on the clinical safety needs and priority needs designated by the patient. We describe how to match these needs to treatment options later in this chapter. Be sure to consider the financial resources that are available to the patient. For example, it is important to know what type of insurance coverage your patient has in case private-pay treatment is not an option.

BRENDA VISITS

It should be clear that in most cases you are the primary clinician and will provide BRENDA visits over the course of treatment regardless of other treatment services that may be required. To this end, you will need to keep an account of other treatments or support groups in which your patient is involved during the time period he or she is seeing you in order to have a full, documented picture of the complete care of your patient. As previously discussed, the frequency of your BRENDA visits will depend upon how many services you are trained to provide, the individual needs of the patient, and the intensity of other services the patient is engaged in as well. Other services may require a large time commitment, reducing his or her availability to meet with you. However, to maintain continuity, we recommend that, unless the patient is in an intensive treatment program, you see the patient weekly for at least the first 3 months, at which time you would likely taper to every other week for the next 3 months, and then monthly for the next 6–12 months of treatment. Even after a treatment episode is successfully completed, it is reasonable to schedule ongoing follow-up visits at 3- and 6-month intervals.

We also recommend that, if you have the training, you provide as much of the treatment as possible that the patient may require. However, freely refer patients for needed services in an area that is outside of your specialty. Try to keep track of these services and coordinate with other treatment providers, if possible.

MEETING SAFETY NEEDS

Someone who comes for treatment and reports drinking large quantities of alcohol and/or has a history of withdrawal symptoms should first receive medical detoxification. As part of your biopsychosocial evaluation, you should have identified those patients who need a medical detoxification before they can begin considering other recovery plans. A medical detoxification can be done on an inpatient or outpatient basis. Our experience shows that the vast majority of alcoholic patients can de detoxified in an outpatient setting. However, inpatient treatment is recommended for very severely dependent alcohol patients, or for those patients who also abuse sedatives, such as high doses of barbiturates or benzodiazepines, where there is a physical danger from seizures or withdrawal delirium that can result in death.

In addition to medical conditions, behavioral and psychological symptoms may also demand immediate attention. For example, symptoms of suicidal or homicidal behavior need to be addressed aggressively and may require immediate inpatient admission. Patients with impaired consciousness, delusions, hallucinations, or paranoid ideation resulting from drug withdrawal, drug intoxication, or serious mental illness are also candidates for inpatient referrals. Safety concerns also extend to a safe environment in which treatment can begin. This includes safety from an abusive family member and a healthy environment of adequate food and shelter. In general, if there is concern about a medical or psychosocial emergency, a referral to an inpatient treatment facility is recommended.

MEETING PATIENT NEEDS

The following is a brief list of the most common types of addiction treatment programs. Some treatment options may not be available in your area.

Behavioral Treatment Options

Inpatient and Outpatient Minnesota Model/12-Step Rehabilitation

The majority of the formal addiction treatment programs across the United States primarily follow the 12-step philosophy and are often called "12-step programs." The 12-step programs tend to work best for patients who are not adverse to total abstinence, and who have a solid employment history and good family support. In the 12-step/disease model, recovery focuses on the patient's acceptance that he or she has a lifelong, biologically driven disease that results in a loss of control in his or her use of alcohol or other drugs. The ultimate way to address this disease is sobriety and total abstinence from these substances. The 12-step model focuses on breaking through denial, providing education about the disease of alcoholism, and moving patients through the 12 steps in order to live without alcohol or drugs. Relapse prevention techniques are also taught. Formalized programs tend to involve spouses, children, and extended families, and there is a strong emphasis on attending mutual-support groups.

Historically, the Minnesota model/12-step programs were set up as residential or inpatient facilities for at least 28 days. This allowed patients to experience an extended period of abstinence and to focus fully on their recovery, away from the natural cues and temptations associated with alcohol and drug use in their environment. Patients with similar problems lived, socialized, and participated in daily treatment together. At discharge, some continued with outpatient treatment, but all were encouraged to continue with regular attendance at AA support groups.

With the introduction in the last decade of managed care into the U.S. health system, current length of inpatient stays are brief (i.e., between 7 and 10 days) and primarily serve the purpose of providing medical stabilization, comprehensive evaluation, and referral to intensive outpatient treatment. Increasingly, even these brief inpatient stays are being eliminated and replaced by intensive outpatient programs (IOPs). The intensity of these programs varies from 3 to 6 hours per day or even every other day. Treatment consists primarily of group therapy and educational lectures and films, with some modest amount of individual addiction counseling. The philosophy of care in these programs is typically AA/12-step based, and attendance at AA or Narcotics Anonymous (NA) meetings outside of formal therapy is strongly recommended.

Typically, an initial IOP treatment course will run for several months. In selecting a program, "more is better" is not always the right option. For patients who have full-time jobs and live a good distance away, a highly intensive program that demands many hours of their time may discourage them from choosing treatment at this time. On the other hand, it is unfortunate, but in today's health care climate, the intensity of the treatment program selected for patients is almost always dictated by the extent of their insurance coverage for alcohol and drug treatment.

Of note, while the 12-step model of recovery is by far the most prevalent and widely recognized method, do not assume that all addiction specialty programs or counselors practice or support the 12-step philosophy. At the same time, there is no gold standard for what philosophy should be followed in addiction programs or outpatient counseling. In fact, there are some well-established, successful addiction programs that do not use the 12-step philosophy but, rather, may follow the principles of cognitive-behavioral therapy, motivational enhancement principles, or a combination of both. While less common, some programs do not have total abstinence as the goal. For example, some localities may have outpatient counselors who support Martha Sanchez-Craig's Drink-Wise program, which supports drinking in moderation. Finally, the quality control of addiction treatment is limited. Assume that some of the addiction-specialized programs and counselors are far more experienced than others. Unfortunately, unless you have personal knowledge of the program or staff, there is really no way to know which are the better-quality programs.

Therapeutic Communities

Therapeutic communities are primarily for persons with illicit drug dependence (primarily cocaine and heroin), who require an intensive program to change. These communities are actually best suited to men with long criminal histories, who are willing to undergo a strong degree of confrontation in order to end their drug habits. The philosophy entails that patients need to be stripped of their rebellious identity before they can be rebuilt as law-abiding citizens. These programs are residential, and the initial treatment is approximately 18 months.

Halfway Houses

These are essentially places where groups of recovering people, who have completed (or are completing) formal rehabilitation programs, live together, with a support staff of counselors available. They are recommended for persons who feel they need to remove themselves from their former living environment in order to maintain abstinence. There are also halfway houses with programs called Oxford Houses, where patients live together without professional support and follow the 12-step philosophy.

Moderation Management

Started in 1995 by Audrey Kishline, this program supports people who are trying to cut down on drinking rather than quit. This program, however, is not for those with serious alcohol dependence or who want to take illicit drugs in moderation. Because it is new, groups may not be available everywhere, but there are now Internet groups devoted to it, and those interested may also get support from several books (i.e., Michael & Jones, 1999).

Cognitive-Behavioral Therapy

Cognitive-behavioral therapy for addiction is based on learning theories of addiction and teaches patients to cope with high-risk situations for relapse with a variety of behavioral and cognitive strategies. These strategies include social reinforcement of abstinent behaviors, cognitive restructuring, learning to cope with environmental cues that elicit craving, and learning behavioral skills to refuse drinks or drug use despite social pressure. Typically, therapy is carried out in individual sessions but can be adapted for groups. This type of addiction treatment has been extensively studied in research settings and can easily be integrated with the use of medications to treat addiction (Irvin, Bowers, et al., 1999).

Mutual Self-Help Groups

Joining a support group is a way for a patient to get continual (daily, if necessary) encouragement while making hard decisions and life changes. Support groups also offer a social network, which can be extremely important, since many people have to stop seeing their drinking and drug-using friends when they quit. Finally, after treatment has been completed, attending support groups can be a cost-free way to continue to derive therapeutic benefits and prevent relapse. Depending on the number of substance-dependent patients you are seeing, you may want to set up groups within your own program that can support each other in their recovery plans.

Alcoholics Anonymous and Other 12-Step Groups

AA is the grandfather of the 12-step movement, and in most U.S. cities, there are meetings available every day. AA is useful for anyone who wants support with abstinence. AA requires nothing of its members but "a desire to stop drinking." It is widely believed that AA is more or less the "standard" for support. There are many variations of AA groups: women only, "double-trouble" (alcohol and psychiatric problems), nonspiritual, nonsmoking, and so on. Also, other 12-step programs include NA, Cocaine Anonymous (CA), and Marijuana Addicts Anonymous (MAA). In some cities, the AA and NA cultures are very different, and some patients with drinking problems may actually find NA more comfortable for them, while some patients with primarily drug problems may find a better home in AA. Therefore, you may need to urge patients to sample several types of groups and locations before deciding whether to reject this option. Have easily accessible copies of an annotated guide of the locations and types of AA meetings in your area to provide your patients.

Patients who take medication for their substance dependence should also be made aware that some 12-step members have a negative attitude toward medications and may try to discourage them from taking their prescribed medications. In the case of comorbidity, there is a pamphlet you can supply to the patient, *The AA Member–Medications and Other Drugs,* that gives AA's actual view on this subject.

Church Groups

Some churches, particularly in the African American community, offer recovery programs that can be very effective, particularly for those who already have ties to a particular church. They tend to use principles similar to those of AA and NA, however, with a more Christian and sometimes a more political activist perspective.

Secular Organization for Sobriety; Women for Sobriety

The Secular Organization for Sobriety and Women for Sobriety are offshoots of AA, with some fundamental differences. The Secular Organization for Sobriety focuses on nonreligious recovery. Women for Sobriety takes a feminist perspective and is only open to women.

Rational Recovery

Rational Recovery is a mutual-support group program for those who want to become abstinent but find the spiritual concepts of the 12-step programs incompatible with the way they think. Rational Recovery members also do not believe that alcohol dependence is a disease and find that after 6 months to a year of abstinence, little further support is necessary. Founded in the late 1980s by Jack Trimpey, and based on the principles of rational emotive therapy, it is widespread, but due to internal disputes, another group, SMART Recovery now also provides a similar program.

SMART Recovery

An offshoot of Rational Recovery, SMART Recovery places less emphasis on founder Jack Trimpey's views. It uses cognitive and behavioral techniques to help members avoid relapse.

Pharmacological Treatments

Methadone Maintenance

This treatment, strictly for opiate addicts, involves the patient taking a daily dose of methadone on an outpatient basis to allay craving and reduce the use of opiates such as heroin. Methadone maintenance has been shown to be effective in reducing both illicit drug use and the spread of infectious diseases such as HIV infections, particularly when methadone maintenance is combined with psychosocial support (McLellan, Arndt, et al., 1993). While effective, the use of methadone maintenance is controversial because patients become physically dependent and will experience withdrawal symptoms if they stop methadone abruptly. Also, because of the risk of illegal diversion, the use of methadone for addiction treatment is restricted to special, approved methadone programs. Since patients taking methadone are required to come to these special programs to receive their daily dose of methadone, patients may feel restricted by the travel. Finally, while most programs offer counseling, continued budgetary cuts have limited the use of these psychosocial services; in some cases, counseling is marginal or no longer in existence.

Patients best suited to methadone maintenance are heroin addicts who have had several treatment failures and are not able to stop opiates entirely. If you are working with patients on methadone and your local methadone program does not provide counseling or support beyond the methadone prescription, you probably will want to refer these patients for additional counseling and encourage them to attend mutual-help groups.

Other Pharmacological Treatments

An important component of treatment from a biopsychosocial model is the integration of medications in the treatment of addiction. Increasingly, the use of medication has been shown to facilitate recovery from alcohol and drug problems, but it does not negate the use of psychosocial treatments. Research shows that the integration of medications such as naltrexone for the treatment of alcoholism with psychosocial support leads to improved treatment outcomes (Volpicelli, Alterman, 1992; O'Malley, Jaffee, et al., 1992). An important difference between the BRENDA approach and other treatment programs is that the use of medications is integrated into treatment rather than being simply tolerated or even actively discouraged.

GIVING DIRECT ADVICE

Having a good sense of the formal and informal, cost and no-cost treatment options in your area allows you to give the most optimal Direct advice to your patients. Again, it is important to emphasize the element of patient choice and the notion that treatment is an option that can help patients improve their lives, not a punishment for "messing up."

Let us look at what you might say to Bill. What options will you suggest to him? Given his willingness to explore changing his drinking habits and his highly visible employment status as a CEO, certain treatment options such as inpatient rehabilitation seem less likely to be a good fit due to social stigma and work commitments. If you suggest this, he will likely decide that you are greatly out of touch with his situation.

CLINICIAN: Your test results indicate that your drinking may be initiating liver damage. I see several ways of proceeding. First, you can try to cut down on your drinking on your own and see if we can get an improvement in your liver enzyme results. If you start experiencing any withdrawal symptoms, I can arrange for you to receive a medical detoxification.

Also, I know at this time you may be concerned about your visibility in the community, but I also want to emphasize that sometimes its "lonely at the top" and support groups can be extremely helpful in maintaining abstinence. Some people in your position seek out support groups in a neighboring county where they are not as likely to run into their neighbors. Also, there are special groups for impaired professionals like yourself. So, if you would like to consider either of these choices, I'm giving you a list of meetings that fit these options. Why not try one out, and we'll talk about it next time we meet?

BILL: I know about AA. I don't want to do that—I don't want to be labeled as an alcoholic.

CLINICIAN: Well, AA is only one of several types of support groups. There is another type, for example, called "SMART Recovery." People who attend these groups also do not want to define themselves as alcoholics or go to meetings for the rest of their lives, but they do want to stop drinking. The rationale is that bad thinking habits keep you drinking when you do not want to, and the focus is therefore on changing these thoughts. They are not religious, and you would attend the group only until you felt you could manage on your own.

BILL: I don't like the idea of telling intimate details of my life to a group of strangers. Can't I just see you or a counselor?

CLINICIAN: That is another option. If you want to see me on a regular basis, we can talk about what I can offer as a treatment option. I can also give you some referrals. There are actually some very good people practicing here.

BILL: Well, I don't know. Will the counseling be about the 12 steps?

CLINICIAN: It sounds as if you are concerned about that approach, which is tied very closely to AA. You could try some cognitive therapies that work very well with drinking problems and are different from the 12-step approach.

BILL: I still can't picture myself talking so much about my problems, but I suppose checking them all out makes sense if I am going to have to do something. Do you think I would have withdrawal?

CLINICIAN: It is hard to say. Individuals vary a great deal. With the amount you say you are drinking daily, it is a possibility, so I would try cutting down for a few days first and see how that goes. I can treat you with a medication if you show signs of severe withdrawal. I could also prescribe a medication for you that will help reduce craving and the chance for a relapse.

BILL: I know that I don't want to take Antabuse.

CLINICIAN: No, I am talking about a medication called naltrexone. It doesn't make you sick if you drink. It just reduces the desire to have a drink, and if you do drink, it reduces the "high" you normally would feel, so you tend to drink less. We have seen excellent results in patients reducing or stopping their drinking by using naltrexone in conjunction with weekly visits with a clinician who is treating their alcohol dependence. Also, naltrexone does not cause physical dependence. If you are interested in this option, I can arrange for you to get a prescription.

BILL: What about side effects?

CLINICIAN: In most cases, there are not any, but as with all drugs, some people do have unpleasant reactions. If you do, we will either reduce the medication dosage or treat the symptoms.

BILL: Well, I might want to try naltrexone. Would I be able to see just you, take my medication, and do all my treatment here?

CLINICIAN: Possibly. However, in some cases we find that a combination of approaches works best. Why don't we take one thing at a time? I am able to prescribe naltrexone, and I will need to monitor your progress on a weekly basis during the course of pharmacotherapy. Our visits would also include discussions about your drinking and life status. As we talk more about this over the course of treatment, if there are other options that could help you while you are seeing me, I can help coordinate other services.

BILL: So if I need to add or change treatments, you would help me with that?

CLINICIAN: Yes, we can work together to make sure that your treatment fits your needs and goals. If you want to change course at any time, it would be up to you, and I would support your decision.

BILL: Well, I think what I'd like to do is first see what the week feels like with me trying to cut down on my drinking. If this doesn't work, then I'd like to try the naltrexone and see you while I'm doing so. Does that seem reasonable?

CLINICIAN: I think it is a very good plan. I would like to see you again next week so that you can let me know how it's going and what you have found out. It would be good if we make the appointment before you leave today, OK? Of course, if you need any other referrals or information before I see you again, please call whenever necessary—particularly if you think you are experiencing withdrawal. I will give you a handout that describes withdrawal symptoms and warning signs that signal you to call me if you haven't already. In some cases, withdrawal symptoms can be dangerous, so no holding back if you get concerned.

BILL: Yes, I'll keep an eye out for withdrawal symptoms, I'll try to cut down on my drinking, and I'll definitely be back next week. Oh . . . I want to think about the support groups. I'm not saying, "No, I won't go ever" but I'm not inclined to do so right now. I have to say that I'm impressed that you recognized my fear of visibility; that is, given my CEO position, I just can't take the chance right now that someone will recognize me. Maybe I'll feel differently someday. Thanks for understanding about this.

CLINICIAN: Bill, let's take one step at a time. And how difficult it is for you to cut back this week will tell us a lot about what kind of changes may or may not be required. OK, see you next week.

As you can see, the advice, offered in a straightforward fashion, provides enough options for the patient to choose his or her own plan. The patient's perspective is fully considered in the resulting plan.

Without going into a full dialogue, here are possible recommendations for an initial plan for Alissa and Stephen.

Alissa

- Inpatient addiction treatment program for 10 days at Center X if her aunt can take her children.

Or

- Intensive addiction outpatient treatment at Center Y, which has free day care.

Or

- Outpatient counseling by a community care provider (possibly using the BRENDA provider), if her aunt can watch the children while she attends treatment.

And

- Pharmacotherapy, including an antidepressant for depression and naltrexone if drinking proves to be a continuing problem. (Refer to physician if you do not have prescribing privileges; refer to a psychiatrist if depression is complicated, persistent, or severe suicidal ideation is present.)

And

- Attend support groups. (Alissa would greatly benefit from support groups, and they do not cost money or require insurance. She needs a lot of support to become abstinent and change her lifestyle, which includes losing her boyfriend. She needs to socialize with healthy, abstinent friends.)

Stephen

- Attend or utilize the Internet to be part of Moderation Management meetings.

And/or

- Cognitive therapy in which there is tolerance for the initial goal of reducing drinking.

And/or

- Naltrexone and referral to a physician for a naltrexone prescription if reduction of drinking fails.

CHAPTER 8

Assessment of the Patient's Reaction to Advice

Adjusting Advice to Patient Response

After 4 weeks of treatment . . .

Bill stopped drinking and began seeing a cognitive therapist once a week. He is taking naltrexone, although at one visit he did not fill his prescription. Bill does not want to attend support groups.

While Alissa has not used cocaine for at least 2 weeks, she does not follow up on any treatment options. She seems more depressed than at her first visit.

Stephen has been attending meetings of Moderation Management. While he has been better at getting to work on time and has had no more accidents, he still binge drinks on weekends and spends a great deal of time thinking about drinking.

RESPONSE TO DIRECT ADVICE: FEEDBACK ON DIRECT ADVICE

Treatment is a process; that is, a prescription or treatment plan is provided, but rarely will you find a patient who adheres to the treatment plan as it was originally formulated. This does not mean that he or she has given up on recovery. Rather, the patient may find some of the plan difficult to follow, or may have developed new notions of what the treatment is about. This is why you want to Assess the patient's reaction to the plan, once tried. This is a good time, also, to dispel patient fears, myths, and concerns, if you can get the patient to voice them. Assessment of the patient's reaction to the Direct advice you gave a week or so ago is an important part of making the BRENDA model work. As always, keeping yourself allied with patients is crucial.

Assessing the Reaction to Direct Advice

The Assessment of the patient's response to advice involves four integrated steps (see Table 8.1). The first step is to conduct a review of the changes in the patient's biopsychosocial evaluation in relation to the last visit and baseline evaluation. Any change in the clinical status between visits provides feedback on the efficacy of the treatment recommendations. Perhaps no other factor helps more to motivate and maintain enthusiasm for following through with treatment recommendations than feedback that one is making progress in treatment. While some visits may be associated with dramatic signs of clinical improvement, there will also be some visits in which the patient appears to have taken a step backward. During these visits, it is important to point out that recovery is not a simple, linear path; it has its cycles of ups and downs. Often, it is helpful to refer back to the baseline clinical state to review the progress made during treatment.

The second step in Assessing the reaction to Direct advice is to compare where the patient is in recovery to his or her goal for recovery. In the early stages of treatment, there may be dramatic improvements in

---

TABLE 8.1. Steps in the Assessment of Response to Direct Advice

1. Assess changes in biopsychosocial status and give positive feedback for any improvements.
2. Compare current status with patient's goal for recovery.
3. Assess whether patient is following up on direct advice and treatment recommendations.
4. Link patient actions (or inaction) on advice to changes in biopsychosocial status (adjust advice if needed).

---

reduction of alcohol and other drug use, but the patient has not achieved a goal of complete abstinence. Just as the treatment of other chronic diseases such as diabetes may not lead to perfect glucose control initially, the first weeks of addiction treatment may not lead to the realization of all the goals of treatment. It is important to note progress toward the goals and use progress to encourage the patient further in treatment. As the patient achieves specific treatment goals, it is helpful to note these accomplishments and give him or her positive feedback. For example, AA has a tradition of marking completion of a set number of abstinent days with a coin to "reward" the individual for achieving an important milestone. In our study with cocaine-dependent mothers, we acknowledge successful completion of 1 month of clean urines with a certificate awarded at a monthly family meeting.

As the third step, assessing response to **D**irect advice includes an assessment of the patient's adherence to the treatment recommendations. Did the patient take all the prescribed medication, attend support groups, follow-through on appointments with other health care providers, and complete any "homework" assignments? Adherence to the treatment recommendations reflects not only the patient's motivation to change but also the quality of the match between the treatment recommendations and the patient's priority needs and other external factors. Often, treatment programs have traditionally assumed that failure to follow a treatment recommendation, such as daily attendance at AA meetings, reflects poor motivation on the patient's part. However, a variety of factors, such as social phobia, poor match with the patient priorities, or even extrinsic factors, such as lack of child care, may contribute to a patient's failure to adhere to treatment recommendations.

In the fourth step, changes in the **B**iopsychosocial assessment are correlated with adherence to the **D**irect advice given at the last visit. So, for example, if the patient who had been drinking a case of beer a day before beginning treatment is now down to drinking three beers on 2 of the last 7 days and has taken all his doses of naltrexone during this time, the clinician notes the correlation between the good medication compliance and the reduction in alcohol use. Conversely, if after several weeks of abstinence, the patient stops taking medication and during the previous week had an episode of alcohol bingeing, the clinician notes the correlation between the medication noncompliance and the return to significant drinking.

The Process of Assessing the Patient Response to Advice

Assessments of the patient's response to your advice should be evaluated following the first visit and at every subsequent BRENDA visit. It is important to remember that the stages of the BRENDA model are touched on at every BRENDA session. Like developmental stages, the emphasis of a particular step depends on the individual patient and his or her stage of recovery. The first sessions may focus on completing a thorough **B**iopsychosocial evaluation, and the second session may focus on **R**eporting the results of the evaluation. Even during these early sessions, you give attention to **E**mpathetic understanding of the patient's perspective, an assessment of safety and personal prioritized **N**eeds, the outlines of the **D**irect advice that you will provide, and the **A**ssessment of how the patient responded to that advice.

HOW TO PRESENT THE ASSESSMENT OF RESPONSE TO DIRECT ADVICE

The **A**ssessment of response to **D**irect advice needs to be integrated into the whole of the BRENDA method. By following the steps—from the initial **B**iopsychosocial evaluation through **R**eporting, **E**mpathetic understanding, **D**irect advice, and **A**ssessment of the patient's reaction to the advice—you create a treatment path that can be adjusted to keep patients motivated on the path of recovery. The examples that follow show how this can be done.

In all three cases, the patients had difficulty following some aspects of the **D**irect advice they had been given. In order to better understand why the "treatment" is not working, it is important to cycle back through the various BRENDA stages. The **B**iopsychosocial evaluation reveals that each patient continues to have problems in some areas. **R**eporting these results in a nonjudgmental, **E**mpathic manner reminds the patient of their **N**eeds, and this sets the stage for further **D**irect advice.

In Bill's case, you can see that he is generally doing well. He has stopped drinking and is getting therapy. But the failure to fill the second naltrexone prescription is cause for concern. It may be that he is headed for relapse, or he may be having side effects. Find out from him what is going on. You do not want to increase resistance, however, so you need to ask him in a way that is as nonaccusatory as possible. The dialogue might proceed like this through the four integrated assessment steps described in Table 8.1.

CLINICIAN: So, how is it going? [**B**iopsychosocial evaluation]

BILL: Well, I have to say I feel a whole lot better since I quit drinking. My wife has stopped nagging me, and I can concentrate better at work. I feel much less tired now. I thought it was just that I was getting older. [Improvement in overall physical health, social interactions with wife, and improved cognitive abilities]

CLINICIAN: That sounds great. When you first came here, you had elevated liver enzymes and the most recent test shows significant improvement, although the levels are still higher than we want to see. Also, you were having problems with your wife complaining about your drinking, and it appears you are getting along better with her now. [Positive feedback from the **R**eport]

BILL: Yeah, and that therapy is much less of a drag than I thought it would be. It's very concrete, and it doesn't take up a whole lot of my time. [Good compliance with one component of the **D**irect advice]

CLINICIAN: I notice that you have not filled your next prescription. Are you having a problem with the naltrexone? [Noncompliance with the medication component of the **D**irect advice]

BILL: No, I was just thinking I do not need to take it any more. I mean, I feel great. I don't want to drink. Why should I keep taking the medication?

CLINICIAN: Well, I can understand your thinking that the medicine is no longer needed. Do you believe the medicine is no longer helping you? [**E**mpathy]

BILL: It really doesn't seem to do much. I couldn't tell anything from it. I just thought, why bother?

CLINICIAN: That makes sense. But if you are not having any side effects, why not take it for the recommended length of time? It certainly is not hurting and it might be helping. [**E**mpathy but also exploring reasons for noncompliance]

BILL: I guess I just didn't want to be dependent on anything, you know?

CLINICIAN: If the medication did not cause dependence, would you take it then?

BILL: No, I would still not want to take it.

CLINICIAN: I noticed that since you started the medication you have had little craving for alcohol and you are moving closer to you goals that we outlined at the beginning of treatment. [Correlating improvement in drinking outcomes with use of the medication] Have your goals changed? [Needs assessment]

BILL: Well, you are right. The medicine appears to be helping me, but I feel so much better now, I guess, in the back of my mind I was wondering if I can have a drink now and then. I don't want to take a pill that is going to block the high from alcohol, although I guess I could finish out the prescription.

CLINICIAN: Well, if you are not having side effects, I don't see why you should stop, especially when you are doing so well. I suspect that if you stopped the medication and had a drink now, you would soon be back to drinking as you were before. The liver is not completely healed and I doubt your wife would be happy if you began drinking again. What do you want to do? [Direct advice and Needs assessment]

BILL: OK, I'll start taking naltrexone again.

Alissa's situation is a bit more difficult. While she has stopped using cocaine, she has not followed through on any advice, has not filled the antidepressant prescription you gave her, and has not checked out any treatment options. After initially refusing, she agreed to an HIV test and was given a referral for the test at the last visit. She seems to be much more depressed than when you last saw her. You are surprised that she has actually shown up for the appointment, but you take this as a sign that somewhere she recognizes that she still needs help. Assessing her situation requires particular gentleness and tact.

CLINICIAN: So, how are you doing? [Biopsychosocial evaluation]

ALISSA: Well, I haven't done coke for 2 weeks.

CLINICIAN: But that's great that you have gone for 2 weeks without using. . . . You should be proud of yourself, because that is a very difficult thing to do. [Positive feedback on abstinence] I received the results of your HIV test and, unfortunately, you are HIV positive. [Report]

ALISSA: I know I'm positive. The testing agency called me a few days ago. What's the point, anyway? I may as well use. I just haven't had the chance to buy yet.

CLINICIAN: I can understand why you feel so discouraged. If you assume that HIV is always fatal, it may seem like there is no use. Fortunately, there is hope with new medications. People are living longer and more normal lives. [**E**mpathy and giving hope]

ALISSA: Thanks, I feel you understand me. No one else does.

CLINICIAN: Also, I see you did not use even though you got terrible news, and I am sure you could have found coke last night if you wanted to. Perhaps there is a part of you that wants to stay abstinent? [**N**eeds assessment]

ALISSA: Yeah, I guess that's true.

CLINICIAN: So, it sounds to me like part of you still wants to recover. It also seems to me that you are very depressed. [**N**eeds assessment and further **B**iopsychosocial evaluation]

ALISSA: Well, wouldn't you be?

CLINICIAN: Of course, I would feel down. But there is a difference between sadness and depression. And, there is quite a bit that can be done now for HIV—but you need to be able to fight it, and you won't be able to do that properly until you deal with your depression as well as your drug problem. Let's talk about some of the options available to you, especially taking antidepressant medication. It's not quite as bad as you think. [**E**mpathy and **D**irect advice]

ALISSA: I'm willing to try again and take antidepressant medication.

In this case, it is clear that a life situation—being diagnosed with HIV— has gotten in the way of treatment progress. If you had simply lectured Alissa on not following advice, chances are, you would not have learned what was really the matter and would have lost her before you were able to help her. But since you followed her lead, you can now help reframe her options and guide her back toward getting the help she needs. Given the severity of her depression, and the fact she did not follow advice previously, you may want to have someone follow up with Alissa to be sure she is taking her medication. Often, a simple phone call from someone who cares will make the difference between whether or not she gets her prescription filled and takes her medication daily.

Because substance-dependent people are used to feeling almost immediate effects from alcohol or drugs, it is important to let patients know that they will probably not notice any helpful effects from antidepressants for about 2 weeks. Otherwise, these patients are particularly prone to give up quickly on medications that seem to have no effect.

Let us turn now to Stephen. He has complied with an important part of the advice that was given to him; that is, he is participating in Moderation Management and ultimately wants to be able to drink moderately. He also is trying to complete the initial month of abstinence recommended for those starting the program, but he tells you that he is still binge drinking on weekends. These behaviors give way to concerns that more trouble at work may be ahead.

CLINICIAN: So, how are you doing with the Moderation Management program? [**B**iopsychosocial evaluation]

STEPHEN: Well, I've been better at not coming in late to work, although Monday mornings are still a problem.

CLINICIAN: Well, that sounds like progress. Are you adhering to the program's guidelines? [**A**ssessing response to **D**irect advice]

STEPHEN: Most of the time. Weekends are really hard. I can't seem to stop drinking when I'm supposed to, and I wind up much more drunk than I want to be. I also think a lot about drinking, but I think I'm getting better.

CLINICIAN: That's much better than when you first came here for treatment. So, are you happy with the progress you have made? [**E**mpathy and **N**eeds assessment]

STEPHEN: Yeah, I'm just a little worried that I get carried away on weekends, but it's better that than giving it all up, I think.

CLINICIAN: Well, if you are still having trouble with this in 2 or 3 more weeks, then we can talk about other options. Perhaps we should consider adding naltrexone or going for complete abstinence as a goal. [**D**irect advice]

STEPHEN: Taking naltrexone might be OK.

From this interview, you can get a sense of Stephen's struggle for control, but you can also see that he is not yet ready to give up drinking. At the next assessment, if he still has not gotten a better handle on it, you will probably have more luck in moving him toward abstinence and other treatment options.

In the next chapter, we look at specific issues related to compliance with medications. Then, in Chapters 10 and 11 we will look at specific issues that may arise in BRENDA visits during the middle and later phases of recovery.

CHAPTER 9

Dealing with Pharmacotherapy
and Medication Compliance Issues

For any medication to be effective, it must be taken regularly. The BRENDA approach is very compatible with helping patients adhere to taking the medication as prescribed as part of the treatment for alcohol or drug dependence (see Pettinati, Volpicelli, et al., 2000). In cycling through the stages of BRENDA, the effective use of pharmacotherapy can be easily integrated. This can be done by (1) providing the patient with education on the specific medication (e.g., how it works, potential side effects; see Appendix B), (2) instilling repeated vigilance in pill taking by regularly asking about it or monitoring pill counts at each visit, and (3) proactively addressing patient issues of medication adherence (i.e., giving advice on individualizing strategies patients can use to combat skipping doses or stopping pill taking; see "Medication Tips for Patients" in Appendix B).

Noncompliance with medication is common throughout medical practice; it is not just a problem among patients on psychotropic drugs. As anyone who has ever prescribed antibiotics knows, patients commonly stop the drugs as soon as the infection is visibly cleared or the pain has ended—despite instructions to take all the medication prescribed.

With respect to medication compliance or adherence, most people do not realize that in *all physical and mental illness*, many people will skip doses or prematurely stop taking their medications. This occurs for a variety of reasons. Thus, part of the pharmacotherapy needs to include an intervention that proactively assists patients in adhering to their daily medication regimen.

It is intuitive, but always good to remind patients that the medication only helps if they take it as prescribed. When a medication fails, most clinicians forget to ask if patients have been taking all of their pills. Thus, it is important to ask about medication compliance in the **A**ssessment of the patient's reaction to **D**irect advice and, when medications are not taken as prescribed, to understand the reasons for missed doses and incorporate suggestions into the **D**irect advice you provide patients.

As discussed, high levels of motivation are the best predictor of medication compliance. But there are times when it is easier for patients to decide to stop taking their pills than to continue their regimen. To address these situations successfully with patients, it is first important to know their attitudes and prior experiences with regular pill taking. For those who are inexperienced or have continually failed at regular pill taking, you will need to spend more time discussing strategies, monitoring pill taking, and so on, during each of the BRENDA visits. While education about the medication is always helpful, if you bring up the topic at each visit for the purpose of determining the status of their pill taking, patients soon realize the importance of taking their pills. Second, it is important to familiarize yourself with the many reasons people skip doses or prematurely stop taking pills. This will help you anticipate adherence issues with your patients before they have had a chance to arise. We summarize below the reasons why patients may stop pharmacotherapy.

DENIAL OF DISORDER

One key reason for noncompliance is denial that there is a problem. With a patient who has decided that he or she does not need the medication or is "cured" prematurely, education is the most helpful technique. Discuss the length of time it can take for the medication to have an effect, and how long a course of treatment may take. Explain that feeling ready to stop treatment before it has gone on long enough to work is common with all illnesses—but as with antibiotics if stopped too soon, there can be worse problems later. Why not be safe, unless other reasons are really behind the desire to stop medication?

Because denial may arise at any time during treatment, education about the disorder and the expectations of the treatment needs to occur throughout the course of care—not just in the early stages. Patients who initially comply may decide to stop taking their medications because they feel that the problem has been treated. They make this decision on their own, without consulting their medical practitioner, and, typically, in the absence of knowledge about relapse rates or other reasons why continuing medication may be necessary.

If you suspect denial, ask questions in a straightforward and nonjudgmental fashion in order to prevent patient resistance. Often, if you are matter-of-fact and nonaccusatory, the real reasons why the patient avoids taking medication will become clear. Ask how they feel about the medication, if they have any fears about it, and what strategies they are using to remember to take it. If they do not have a set routine and need a way to develop one, see the section "Forgetting to Take Medications" later in this chapter and "Medication Tips for Patients" in Appendix B.

If patients express doubt that the condition is serious enough to warrant medication treatment, gently but continually remind them of their presenting symptoms and of the past consequences of their drug and alcohol use (again, the BRENDA Report). Emphasize the fact that having an alcohol dependence problem is not the patients' fault, but also stress their responsibility for getting treatment and properly following treatment instructions.

Another way of handling this problem is to emphasize the use of medication as an "aid" rather than as a sign of the severity of the problem.

Be sure that you are actually dealing with denial. Other reasons such as simple forgetting and a failure to establish a consistent strategy to remember medication may seem similar. Because of this, it is important to determine proactively the patient's history of medication compliance in other circumstances. If he or she has never taken medication consistently, it is likely that these issues, rather than denial, are paramount.

DEFICITS IN KNOWLEDGE

Noncompliance with medication can also result when patients have false beliefs about what the medication will and will not do. For example, patients on antidepressants may quickly decide that the pills are worthless if they were not warned that it takes about 2 weeks or more before they notice any changes in their mood.

Naltrexone's primary effect is to reduce cravings, and reduce the desire to drink more after slips. This may make it difficult for patients to know early on whether it is helping and may be particularly prominent if patients have no side effects and "feel nothing" when they take the medication. To combat this, inform patients that they may not know when the drug has taken effect, but that over time, they will see a change in their drinking behavior.

Persons with substance dependence are particularly prone to wanting instant effects from their medications. Warn patients that naltrexone or other "antidrug" pharmacotherapy does not work like this. Thoroughly discuss their expectations so that you know their beliefs. Use every opportunity to correct false ideas about what the medication will and will not do.

Additionally, some patients who return to drinking may see this as a failure of medication. Let them know that this is not necessarily so—that the drug will help reduce continued drinking even if they have already taken one drink, and that one or two "slips" do not indicate treatment failure or relapse. Inform them of Prochaska and DiClemente's (1983) research on quitting smoking, which shows that the more times a person tries quitting, the more likely he or she will eventually succeed.

There is another important knowledge deficit that must be combated as well. Patients with substance dependence may have overly simplistic ideas about how drugs interact with neural pleasure systems. They might refuse or stop naltrexone because they fear that it will prevent them from experiencing any positive feelings or natural highs.

While it is true that naltrexone can sometimes block "runner's high" and the high experienced by some people after eating spicy foods, it certainly does not, in most people, eliminate pleasure. The brain is much more sophisticated than this, with several different systems for positive reinforcement, only one of which is opiate-mediated. Of course, if anhedonia does occur, and seems linked to naltrexone then the medication should be discontinued, because anhedonia is a strong trigger for relapse. These issues should be discussed openly and honestly with the patient. A patient is much more likely to be compliant if he or she knows that you are not trying to take away the fun in life and respect the natural human desire for pleasure.

UNCOMFORTABLE SIDE EFFECTS

Of course, patients will wish to stop any medication that they associate with unpleasant side effects. Although it would seem logical that this would be the most important reason why people might stop taking medications, this appears not to be the case with naltrexone. In fact, in two studies done at the University of Pennsylvania, the patients reporting the most side effects with naltrexone were not the ones most likely to drop out of outpatient treatment. This is not to say that side effects are unimportant, but framing them properly can greatly improve medication adherence.

Specifically, the most important thing is to help patients determine whether their reported adverse experiences are actually linked to the medication or to other factors in their lives. For example, many patients who have just quit using drugs and alcohol experience anxiety; if they are taking a medication, they might logically feel that their anxiety is due to this. Looking at the entire situation is important. Clearly, if the anxiety persists and does seem linked with the medication, a reduction in dose would be in order. This way, the patient may decide if there is a connection on his or her own. If lowering the dose does not result in any change, look for other causes. The severity and "annoyance" of side effects should also be discussed. One patient may find a side effect unbearable, while another might see it as simply bothersome. Talk through the pros and cons of continuing medication; some patients might find that the benefits outweigh the annoyance, while others might have to discontinue the treatment.

If there occurs a serious adverse experience that may be related to the medication, it should be discontinued immediately, and there are reporting requirements to the U.S. Food and Drug Administration and pharmaceutical companies that must be followed. If the adverse experience is neither serious nor related to the medication, as mentioned earlier, it is important to discuss alternate explanations with patients, as this often alleviates their concern and helps them stay in treatment. When a decision is made to discontinue treatment, the clinician will want to feel sure that the reason for doing so has been fully explored and tested.

Sometimes the patient will use side effects as an excuse, for example, wanting to stop the medication in order to get "high" again. Ask the patient directly about the impact of the side effects on his or her life versus the impact of a potential relapse, and whether he or she is missing the feeling of getting high. As always, do not become accusatory or create the impression that you want the patient to take medications at all costs. The patient needs an empathetic ear at this point. However, it is your responsibility to help the patient find reasons to continue treatment if possible.

A DESIRE TO GET HIGH

Some patients will likely discontinue medications because they want to drink or get high again. As with dealing with denial, you want to be nonjudgmental when discussing urges to use. Stress that these urges are normal, and that they will pass. Talk about why the patient wants to drink or take drugs, and what alternate activities might be considered. Discuss the possible impact of a return to active addiction, and the effect that alcoholism might have on the areas of life that the patient has said are most important; ask what else might be done to help. Remember, if the patient believes you want him or her to enjoy life and that treatment is not meant to be punitive, he or she is much more likely to stick with the program.

Be on particular guard for anhedonia and depression. If a patient feels that nothing but getting high will offer relief and joy, you need to be sure that there is not a chemical reason why normal life activities are not satisfying. If anhedonia is present (and not naltrexone-dose related), discuss a course of antidepressants to relieve it.

LACK OF CONTROL OVER A CHAOTIC LIFE

If someone is living with an abusive partner who deals drugs, has seven children and does not work, it is likely that he or she may not have enough structure or control to do anything consistently, particularly taking medication. It is advisable to get such patients started in a structured, daily outpatient program *prior* to starting medication (or refer them for inpatient treatment if possible, followed by outpatient treatment). This way, the medication can become part of their newly structured lives; then, as they gain the ability to create their own structure, the medication regimen is already established.

Of course, people vary greatly in chaotic situations; some persons who are very motivated to change may be able to create structure in situations where they were not previously in control, while others may not. Be careful not to overgeneralize.

FORGETTING TO TAKE MEDICATIONS

Even people with life-threatening diseases often forget to take their medications. While this may be a consequence of denial, it can also be related to the fact that the human memory is far from perfect. It is not unusual for patients to get caught up in the details of living and forget to take a dose of medication, or forget that they have already taken their dose for the day.

Research indicates that complicated medication regimens and lengthy periods of treatment negatively correlate with medication compliance rates (Salzman, 1995). Studies also have revealed that patients are more likely to comply with medication instructions on days immediately before and after seeing their clinicians (Cramer, Scheyer, et al., 1990).

There are several logical, commonsense ways to combat forgetfulness, but we should not assume that patients will develop these strategies on their own. Once it is established that the patient is actually forgetting (i.e., not making an excuse because of denial, embarrassing side effects, etc.), a clinician can take steps to teach techniques that aid memory.

First, discuss the patient's lifestyle and circumstances, and the types of routines he or she performs daily. Ask if he or she takes vitamins or other medications routinely, and how (and whether) he or she remembers to take them. If the patient has a successful routine, see if he or she can incorporate the treatment medications into it. If there is no established routine, before devising one, ask if the patient used one for any pill taking in the past.

If the patient has little to no experience or has been unsuccessful with pill taking, ask if there is anything—such as eating breakfast, having a morning cup of coffee, brushing teeth, watching a particular television show—that he or she does daily without fail. Try making the medication part of that ritual—if need be, suggest initially posting a note or reminder, until taking the medication becomes a daily habit.

Other techniques to help a patient remember to take medications involve asking a significant other to help out (but only if "nagging" or power struggles in the relationship are not an issue) or getting a pill dispenser that beeps at the appropriate time. If possible, calling the patient between visits can also be helpful—as can decreasing the time between visits. Patients tend to comply best with pill taking immediately before and after medical visits, and a phone call can have a similar effect.

Some patients may not only forget to take medications, but may also forget whether they have taken them. To avoid this, try to get medications packaged in a daily blister pack, or use a pillbox with pockets for each particular day. Sometimes the simplest and most obvious technique, such as placing the pills at eye level in open view (but out of the reach of young children) and not away in a cabinet, can make a big difference. Some memory aids that may be helpful to patients are described in "Medication Tips for Patients" in Appendix B.

LOST MEDICATIONS/FAILURE TO RENEW PRESCRIPTIONS

Another reason for lack of medication compliance is that patients may lose medication or fail to renew a prescription. To deal with these problems, make sure you let patients know that they can renew their prescription at any time, and that you will always be available to change a prescription or replace lost medication.

To prevent loss, patients should place this prescription with other medications or vitamins that they regularly take; keeping it in the same place consistently. Advise them to renew prescriptions at least a week in advance, so that there is no opportunity for missed medication.

Indigent patients who must pay directly for their medication may not be able to afford the prescription at certain times, and steps should be taken to assure that lack of money does not interfere with treatment continuity.

█████

CHAPTER 10

Applying the BRENDA Stages to Early Recovery Issues

After 9 weeks of treatment . . .

Bill did continue the naltrexone, but he took one drink at his daughter's wedding. Realizing that he might be headed for trouble, he did not continue drinking, but he mentions it anxiously when you see him.

Alissa's mood has improved on antidepressants. She has been living with her aunt and consistently attends her BRENDA visits and NA support groups, but she is frightened because she will soon have to return home.

Stephen has continued with Moderation Management and seemed to be doing better until last week, when he missed a day at work because he was too hung over to go in. He is now better able to discuss other treatment options.

Following detoxification/stabilization, patients enter the early recovery phase, which typically runs through the first 6 months of treatment. In these examples, the patients have made substantial progress, yet each is dealing with common early recovery issues. During this early recovery phase, the chance of a relapse to excessive and destructive drinking or drug use is high. It is often disappointing for patients to realize that even after a month of continuous sobriety they still feel foggy or not quite right. As the patient experiences exposure to alcohol and other drugs at social functions and is confronted with well-meaning invitations to share a drink or take a hit on the coke pipe, the temptation to use can be overwhelmingly high. The pain of the factors that originally brought the patient into treatment may no longer be present, thus reducing his or her motivation to continue with treatment.

In order to support the patient during the early recovery phase, continue to follow the basic BRENDA stages. While the comprehensive **B**iopsychosocial evaluation does not need to be repeated at each visit, continual monitoring and assessment of the original problems should occur at each visit during early recovery. Also, screen for any new problems, such as changes in physical health, mood, or social interactions. Ironically, many patients only recognize other chronic medical problems once they become sober. Also, feelings of emptiness or even full-blown depression accompany the loss of their special "love" for their drug of abuse. Even social relationships undergo dramatic and not always pleasant evolutions, as a spouse may, paradoxically, react negatively to the patient's newfound sobriety.

It is a good idea to know what problems patients are facing, so that you can provide support by reinforcing positive behaviors. In your sessions, you will also be monitoring patients' progress and adjusting your advice according to their changing needs and growth. These will vary in accordance with their stage of recovery (e.g., suggestions that may work in the early stages may not be appropriate for patients who are further along). As treatment progresses, responsibility for change is increasingly transferred from the clinician to the patient. For example, someone experiencing DTs cannot be expected to responsibly search for a job. As recovery progresses, however, increasing responsibility is placed on patients to manage their needs. In the early phase of recovery, however, the clinician is still quite active in managing patients' programs of recovery.

Table 10.1 lists issues that commonly need attention during early recovery. We have already touched on other medical problems and difficulties that may arise in family and social interactions. The balance of this chapter looks at dealing with protracted withdrawal symptoms, risk of relapse, employment, sexual activity, and partner issues.

TABLE 10.1. Early Recovery Issues

- Protracted withdrawal symptoms
- Attention to other medical problems
- Increased risk of relapse to destructive drug use
- Social interactions
- Family issues
- Sexual activity
- Employment

PROTRACTED WITHDRAWAL SYMPTOMS

In early recovery, patients have to contend with the problem of persistent withdrawal symptoms. While most of these do resolve in the first 2 weeks or so of abstinence, irritability, mood swings, and sleeplessness (particularly in alcohol and opiate dependence) can last for months during an initial period of abstinence. It is important to let patients know that although these symptoms may last quite a while, they will eventually pass and recovery will become more comfortable for them. Otherwise, they are likely to think that they will always remain in an unpleasant state. If patients truly believe that the state is long-lasting, relapse will occur because it brings some pleasure.

Life without pleasure is certainly a huge relapse trigger. Technically called anhedonia, this is a very important withdrawal sign in early abstinence from cocaine, and it can linger for as long as 6 months of abstinence from alcohol or drugs. It can also be a symptom of severe depression. Try to evaluate patients for it by checking their motivations, their pleasurable activities, and their level of joy in life. Thus, for some patients an important need is to address these unpleasant symptoms of protracted withdrawal. If you suspect anhedonia, antidepressant medication may be indicated, because relapse is very common in patients experiencing anhedonia.

THE RELAPSE PROCESS

Patients in early recovery should be taught to recognize that the steps toward lapses and relapses often begin long before the actual drink or drug is consumed. Triggers are part of this process—whether emotional situations, physical sensations, or "people, places, and things." Learning how to recognize whether they are heading for danger is an important skill that patients in early recovery need to master.

Identifying the Needs behind Triggers

Everyone has certain situations that make them uncomfortable, and when people with alcohol and drug dependence feel uncomfortable, they tend to think first of taking a drink or using a drug to ease these feelings. Much of lapse and relapse prevention revolves around identifying these "trigger" situations and either avoiding them or finding better ways of coping with the discomfort they evoke. In the very early stages of quitting drugs and alcohol, avoidance is best. But if the patient cannot progress beyond that, recovery is doomed to fail because sooner or later everyone has to confront uncomfortable feelings.

In Bill's case, being at his daughter's wedding, with his ex-wife and present wife both in attendance, was certainly a trigger-type situation. Bill not only had to deal with all the emotions of his eldest daughter's marriage, but also he had to deal with the conflicts between his two families in a situation where alcohol was widely available.

In order to prevent his lapse from recurring, it is important to help him realize what exactly pushed him over the edge into actually taking the drink. The dialogue might go something like this.

BILL: I screwed up. I knew I shouldn't have taken that drink, but everyone was making a toast and I just felt like I couldn't refuse a glass of champagne. As soon as I tasted it, I knew it was a mistake. And my daughter gave me such a look—she knew I wasn't supposed to be drinking, and she'd been so proud that I wasn't drunk for her wedding.

CLINICIAN: In the past, when you drank at a social function, you would have at least six drinks and get drunk, yet this time you didn't get drunk, did you? [**R**eporting back to the patient]

BILL: No, it was strange. I guess that stuff must be working because I didn't want any more. Normally, once I'd had one glass, all bets would be off.

CLINICIAN: Let's talk about why you felt you had to drink. If we can figure that out, I think you can avoid having this happening again in similar situations. [Trying to identify what N̲eed triggered a desire to drink]

BILL: Well, hopefully, she's not going to get married again!

CLINICIAN: Yes, but what was the feeling you had right before you gave in to the urge to drink?

BILL: I don't know. Well, I guess I was thinking that I was the only one there who wouldn't be having a drink, and I was thinking that people would think I was an alcoholic if I didn't have one. I guess I thought about my daughter when she was little, and how she was all grown up now, and it all sort of . . . I didn't want to think about it and I thought one drink couldn't hurt . . .

CLINICIAN: So, you didn't want to feel what you were feeling, and you were in a situation where you felt social pressure to drink? [N̲eed to appear social at function in which others are drinking]

BILL: Yeah, you could put it that way.

CLINICIAN: Well, what if you thought about the situation ahead of time? For example, a big family event like a wedding is bound to be emotionally stimulating. So knowing that, you could make plans to either have a nonalcoholic beverage on hand for toasts, for example, or have someone available you can call to talk about your feelings if you start having an urge to drink. You can also always leave a situation where you feel uncomfortable and, for example, go to the men's room until the feeling passes. Or even just eat something—many times that also helps. [Giving D̲irect advice]

BILL: Yeah, I guess I just didn't think about it—I thought it would be a happy event.

CLINICIAN: Sometimes happy events are as dangerous as upsetting events for triggering drinking.

Learning to Protect against Triggers

As you can see, on the one hand, Bill unwittingly put himself in a situation where he endangered his recovery. On the other hand, he could not have avoided his own daughter's wedding. However, he could have anticipated a wedding toast and planned how he would handle it. In order to prevent relapse, it is necessary to get the patient to think about what situations (people, places, and things) most strongly provoke the desire to drink or use drugs. You then either suggest that the patient avoid them or learn to protect him- or herself when encountering these situations.

Some situations that trigger relapse are obvious—entering a crack house when you are trying to quit crack cocaine makes little sense, as does hanging out with crack cocaine addicts. But some situations are subtler. Bill's wife may have been nagging him not to drink, but the dynamics that developed in his relationship with her may have made some of the things she said act as a trigger for his drinking, even though she herself does not imbibe. Someone that the patient loves and respects, who has continually advocated for the patient to quit, may be a trigger because the fear of failing to please him or her is so great. Because of this, it is important that patients talk about the emotions and situations that immediately preceded their worst binges and come to understand which circumstances are most likely to lead to relapse.

Alissa, for example, knows that her apartment, where she did most of her drinking and crack cocaine smoking, is a trigger for her. She knows that her drug-dealer boyfriend is someone she should avoid. But she has to move back to her place as her inpatient treatment ends because she can no longer impose on her aunt to watch her children. She believes he has moved out but is fearful of all of the triggers in her house.

Let us look at some suggestions that might be given to her for dealing with the situation.

ALISSA: I wish I didn't have to go back there. Everything in that place reminds me of crack.

CLINICIAN: Yes. But you don't have to go back to getting high. One thing that might help is rearranging your furniture. [Giving **D**irect advice]

ALISSA: What?

CLINICIAN: Well, if you do that, it will remind you that things have changed, and you don't get high anymore. Also, have you arranged for your sponsor from NA to come with you when you move? [More **D**irect advice]

ALISSA: Nah, I told her I could manage.

CLINICIAN: I know you may feel that you can and should be able to manage on your own. [Empathy] However, you might want to rethink that. You don't know how you'll feel when you open the door. If someone who's clean is there, you are much less likely to pick up. [More Direct advice]

As you can see, the clinician makes concrete suggestions for dealing with these situations, and helps the patient think them through.

Common Triggers (HALT)

The collective wisdom of the 12-step programs has identified another common group of triggers, which are easily remembered by the acronym HALT—Hungry, Angry, Lonely, and Tired (see Table 10.2). Each of these feelings can push someone toward a drink or a drug. Hunger and tiredness are often not obvious because alcohol and drugs have distorted the human metabolism. Patients with substance dependence often are out of touch with their bodies' needs and interpret any discomfort as desire for alcohol or a drug. They are often amazed at how eating or sleeping resolves bad moods when they are hungry or overly tired. In these cases, the solutions are obvious: sleep or eat.

For anger and loneliness, calling a friend in recovery, or just someone who will be supportive is recommended. This can be a hard habit to form for those who are not used to reaching out; however, it is very useful in preventing slips. You may want to match up patients who are in recovery together so that they can create a network to support each other in these situations, or you may want to have a staff person on a beeper to take their phone calls.

When social support is not enough to reduce unpleasant feelings,

TABLE 10.2. The HALT Common Triggers

Trigger		Coping response
H	Hungry	Eat
A	Angry/anxious	Call a time-out to relax
L	Lonely	Call a supportive friend
T	Tired	Sleep

individual therapy may be a useful adjunct. For primary care providers, referrals to clinicians with a mental health background are an option. For mental health professionals, Needs can be addressed in the individual BRENDA sessions. Remember, the BRENDA model can be a team approach; you are not expected to have all the answers or provide all aspects of treatment. When triggers indicate a Need that is outside your area of expertise, you should consider a referral to an appropriate clinician.

Distinguishing between Lapse and Relapse

Although 12-step model treatments consider any use of drugs or alcohol a relapse, other models make a distinction between a "lapse" or "slip" and a full-fledged "relapse." This distinction is useful because there can be more shame attached to relapse than a slip.

In order to prevent inordinate negative consequences from an "abstinence violation," the notion of a lapse or slip was developed. A lapse or slip can be a warning that a patient is heading in the wrong direction, but it does not have to mean that he or she has arrived at a dead end; that is, a lapse is an error that can be corrected before serious consequences occur. The chances of irreparable damage to a patient's job, social relationships, and personal reputation are far more likely with a relapse than with a lapse. However, even should a total relapse occur, it could be reframed as a learning experience.

It is particularly useful to make this distinction in the course of naltrexone treatment, since the drug can help prevent a lapse from becoming a relapse, and patients should, of course, be informed that naltrexone has this ability. When lapses or relapses occur, you will want to explore the circumstances that led up to it very thoroughly with your patients. The more patients can identify the things that precede and push them into a drinking or drug use situation, the more likely they will be able to avoid future relapses.

Lapse and Relapse in Moderation Management

Because some drinking is allowed in programs where the goal is moderation, "relapse" is defined as drinking more than your limit for that particular day.

Stephen not only has reported a consistent struggle with remaining at his drinking limit, but the times when he has gone over the limit, there were serious consequences for him, such as putting his job in jeopardy. It is time to talk to him about other possible ways of dealing with his problem.

CLINICIAN: So, how are you progressing with your plan to control your drinking? [**B**iopsychosocial evaluation]

STEPHEN: I did it again. Drinking moderately is much harder than I thought it would be. I really thought I could manage it, but every weekend it seems that I end up drunk. I can't believe I am being so stupid.

CLINICIAN: Do you know why you drink so much more on weekends? [Attempt to determine **N**eeds]

STEPHEN: Well, once I have two or three, and I can't think of a reason why I shouldn't have more—well, that's it. I lose track. I drink in the morning. I can't stop.

CLINICIAN: So, it sounds like you really are not able to drink moderately.

STEPHEN: No, I guess not. I never realized how much of my life I spend thinking about drinking.

CLINICIAN: Would you like to try something different? [**N**eeds assessment]

STEPHEN: Well, I don't know. I still don't know what I'd do if I had to stop drinking.

CLINICIAN: I have a thought. Why don't you try not to drink for just a brief period, like, say, 2 or 3 months? If you don't like how you feel at the end of this period, I'm sure the bars will still be open. [**D**irect advice]

STEPHEN: I don't know.

CLINICIAN: I can understand why you may feel pessimistic, but what do you have to lose? [**E**mpathy]

STEPHEN: I'm afraid that I won't be able to do it. Over the last 2 weeks, when I was trying to cut down, I could see how much I want to drink.

CLINICIAN: Well, there are ways of getting around that. I'd like you to try a new medication that helps relieve craving for alcohol. [**D**irect advice]

STEPHEN: Wow, that's just what I need. I really don't want to have another weekend like this one.

CLINICIAN: Well, this is not a miracle drug . . . you will still need to try not to drink. However, I think it will make things bearable for you and help you get through the initial period that you are fearful about.

STEPHEN: I'm willing to try this medication, if you think it'll help me think less about drinking.

As you can see, the clinician has helped Stephen see his preoccupation with drinking as part of a larger pattern that points to him having a more serious drinking problems than he first thought. As the clinician encourages him to rethink his goals [patient priority **N**eeds], he moves Stephen toward motivation to change.

Often, a good indicator of potential trouble is a desire not to take naltrexone, when it is not linked to side effects or any other rational reason. For example, just after Stephen started on naltrexone, a female friend invited him to meet her in a bar one evening. Let us explore how this problem might be discussed in a BRENDA session.

CLINICIAN: So, how it is going? Are you having any side effects? [**B**iopsychosocial evaluation]

STEPHEN: No, not really.

CLINICIAN: Did you take the medication today? [**A**ssessing response to **D**irect advice]

STEPHEN: Well, actually, I forgot.

CLINICIAN: Do you think there was any reason why you forgot it today? [**N**eeds assessment]

STEPHEN: No, I can't think of any.

CLINICIAN: Well, it occurs to me that it's Friday.

STEPHEN: Yeah, that's true.

CLINICIAN: And from what you've been telling me, this has normally been a big drinking night for you. [Attempt to determine **N**eeds]

STEPHEN: Yeah, and I'm actually supposed to meet my friend Stacy at a restaurant tonight.

CLINICIAN: So, were you planning on drinking?

STEPHEN: No, I don't think I was. I mean, now that I think of it, it could have been that I had that thought, because I think I'm a little worried about what Stacy will think, and I'm not sure why she wanted to see me alone.

CLINICIAN: Right. So, can you remember what you thought this morning when you decided not to take it?

STEPHEN: You are right. The situation did flash in my mind, and I thought, nah, I'll just take it later, in case I decide I'll be too uncomfortable and need a drink. I put it right out of my mind though, and then I really did forget that I hadn't taken it.

CLINICIAN: That sounds right. This is often how relapse happens—it's very tricky and sneaks up on you.

STEPHEN: You know, I didn't even think about it that way. I just thought, I'll worry about it later. I can handle it.

CLINICIAN: Yes, those are the thoughts that often get people in trouble.

STEPHEN: Yeah, I guess you are right. I guess I should take it now, shouldn't I?

CLINICIAN: Yes, unless you want to wind up having another weekend like the last one. [Direct advice]

STEPHEN: No, you're right. I don't. I guess, like you say, I need to watch my thoughts and not let it catch me like that.

CLINICIAN: It seems to me that in your case, you need to watch particularly for emotional situations—like, where you might feel uncomfortable or unsure of what is expected of you. [Direct advice]

STEPHEN: I guess so. Yeah, you know, I never thought that was why I drank, but I guess the more I think about it, the more it seems this may be why.

Note how the clinician makes sure to address Stephen's particular situation and to point out triggers that are specific for him. It is always important to discuss whether the patient has taken the medication regularly, and to look for the reasons behind any failure to adhere to the medication or any part of the treatment regimen. As preparation, be ready to offer alternate ways of coping with the triggers. In Stephen's case, for example, you might discuss why he wants to keep this date, and propose alternate meeting places that are unrelated to alcohol use.

EMPLOYMENT

For many patients in early recovery, work is of great concern. Some may have taken off time for medical detoxification treatment. Others may feel that their jobs are now more stressful than when they were drinking or using drugs. Still others may have been unemployed and now wish to work, because they need to fill the time they once spent getting high.

Since job satisfaction is linked with long-term recovery, it is important to help patients resolve work issues. In early recovery, recognizing work-related triggers is most important. For the employed, learning to deal with job stresses and frustrations, and to recognize which aspects of work they enjoy and which ones make them uncomfortable (facets that are frequently masked while drinking and drugging), rather than making major and immediate changes, should be encouraged. You should try to leave the resolution of major work issues for later, when the patient has been clean for at least 6 months to a year.

Many people suggest that the unemployed take "recovery jobs" (i.e., simple, easy work that is not challenging but that requires them to get into the habit of showing up every day). This can be useful in building self-esteem and is helpful for those who have not worked for a long time. It also cuts down on time available for impulsive relapses. If paid work is not available, volunteer work can serve much the same purpose.

SEXUAL ACTIVITY AND PARTNER ISSUES

Another area that often causes particular trouble in early recovery is sex. Some men may find themselves impotent due to withdrawal-related changes, and people of both genders may find themselves unused to having sex without drinking or drugs. Furthermore, because sex with a partner often elicits extreme emotions, it is a common trigger for relapse.

Some programs suggest that patients avoid sex (other than masturbation) during their first year of recovery, but many people who have just given up drinking and drugs do not wish to give up sex as well. Since many drug withdrawal syndromes feature increased sex drive, few people manage to follow this suggestion. Given this phenomenon, the best way to deal with the issue is to find patients' areas of discomfort. If they feel that giving up sex for a while may be a relief, then reinforce the suggestion. Notice that the patient's priority need here is to experience relief by not having to deal with sexual issues during recovery. The BRENDA method can support this patient's need by recommending sexual abstinence. On the other hand, some patients feel that sex is very important and wish to be open to possible sexual experiences right away. If that is the patient's priority need, then the clinician can support this and discuss potential problems and how to deal with them prior to the experience, if possible.

Because formal recovery programs that involve group interaction often bring people in close emotional contact, many individuals develop new relationships during recovery. While the camaraderie can engender support and combat loneliness, it can also be a dangerous time both physically and emotionally. Treatment programs try to discourage "rehab romances," and the level of involvement and duration is usually short-term. Nevertheless, they happen. Rather than provoking resistance by disparaging the relationship, try to determine possible trouble areas and work on bolstering immunity to relapse instead. People with alcohol and drug addiction are a high-risk group for HIV and hepatitis. If you think your patient is sexually active, an instruction session on the use of condoms is generally a good idea.

CHAPTER 11

Applying the BRENDA Stages to Later Recovery Issues

Six months after beginning treatment . . .

Bill has now been alcohol-free for 3 months. He is doing well both at work and at home but is tired of his job and the stresses associated with it. He would like to stop taking naltrexone.

Alissa has been drug-free for 5 months and her youngest child is entering kindergarten. She is not quite sure what to do without her kids at home during the day, since they have always required constant attention. She attends an NA meeting every day.

Stephen gave up Moderation Management and began attending AA meetings. With the help of daily naltrexone, he has been almost alcohol-free for about 3 months and feels ready to move on.

Patients with between 3 and 6 months abstinence from compulsive use of drugs and alcohol have generally completed the first phase of recovery. For the most part, their bodies and brains have adjusted to living without alcohol and drugs (or to moderation, if they have done it successfully), and they have made the essential changes in their lifestyle in order to put addiction behind them. At this point, the issues that face them tend to be real-life issues: what to do now that drugs and alcohol no longer play a major role in their lives, and what positive, long-term goals should replace the distraction of addiction. A list of common late recovery issues appears in Table 11.1.

TRIGGERS REVISITED

In early recovery, avoidance of triggers is the safest approach, but in later phases, patients may start to feel limited and unhappy if they are constantly having to turn down invitations to parties where alcohol will be present, or avoid restaurants, dance lounges, rock concerts, and the like. The younger the patient, the more acute these feelings may be. Late recovery involves a reevaluation of how to deal with relapse triggers.

You should monitor your patients' feelings and decisions related to "triggers." If they are comfortable with continuing to avoid these types of situations, do not push. If, however, they want to start returning to a wider social life, you need to explore their motivations. Of course, being in places where alcohol or drugs are available requires a particular vigilance against impulsiveness, and this is often the type of issue discussed in BRENDA sessions at this phase of recovery.

Let us look at how a BRENDA session with Stephen might proceed.

STEPHEN: My friend's band is playing this weekend, and I haven't gone to see them since I've been abstinent. I can't sit around at home anymore . . . I'm going nuts . . .

TABLE 11.1. Later Recovery Issues

- Expanding coping responses for triggers (beyond avoidance)
- Long-standing emotional pain behind the addiction (e.g., childhood issues, abuse)
- Current life issues postponed during early recovery (e.g., employment, life skills)
- Relapse prevention as a long-term process
- When to stop treatment

CLINICIAN: Well, why don't you go hear them?

STEPHEN: Everyone keeps telling me not to see old friends, not to go anywhere that alcohol is served. My girlfriend is dead set against it.

CLINICIAN: Do you think you would drink? [Needs assessment]

STEPHEN: No. I know those guys drink a lot, but I don't want to do that anymore. I would just like to hear the music, have a good time, you know?

CLINICIAN: Let's say you did go. How would you protect yourself if someone offered you a drink?

STEPHEN: I would refuse it, say that I don't do that anymore.

CLINICIAN: Do you feel comfortable doing that?

STEPHEN: Oh, yeah. I mean, I don't care about it. If they tease me, which they do anyway, I'll give it right back.

CLINICIAN: And what if you felt like drinking?

STEPHEN: I just won't.

CLINICIAN: What could you do to prevent it, if you felt the urge?

STEPHEN: Call someone?

CLINICIAN: That's good. Anything else?

STEPHEN: Um . . .

CLINICIAN: Here's an important thing I want you to keep in mind. You can always leave. If the situation is uncomfortable for you, don't worry about being rude or what others will think. Just leave. They can take care of themselves and you can always come up with an explanation later. In fact, be sure that you can always leave these types of situations. Drive there yourself, and if you are going with your girlfriend or someone, explain that you may have to leave if you feel uncomfortable. It is important that they understand and respect this. [Direct advice]

STEPHEN: OK, that makes sense. And I guess I could bring someone who won't drink.

CLINICIAN: Yes, that is always a good idea as well.

CHILDHOOD ISSUES

Patients who are in individual therapy or attend support groups may begin to reflect on their childhood as they progress through the recovery process. In the early stages, most of the focus will be on immediate issues of withdrawal and avoiding relapse. But as that gets further away, emotional pain, which has long gone unheeded, may make itself felt and can lead to relapse if not handled properly.

Since there is much greater incidence of emotional, physical, and sexual abuse in the childhoods of patients with substance dependence (particularly, but not exclusively, women), it is important that practitioners be aware of these issues. If patients raise these issues, be ready to refer them to individual therapists and groups that can help them deal with these matters. Check out the resources in your area with someone you trust before you make referrals, because some fraudulent treatment exists in this area. Some patients may also wish to attend support groups related to these issues. Among the most common are Adult Children of Alcoholics, Al-Anon, and Codependents Anonymous.

LIFE CHANGES REVISITED

Once a patient has been able to maintain months of successful recovery, issues of work and relationships, which were disregarded during the crisis of withdrawal and avoiding relapse, will surface. If recovery is to be maintained, major changes in these areas may need to take place.

For example, unemployed patients are at high risk for relapse. In Alissa's case, the need for work is particularly heightened by the fact that her children are no longer infants. Without their constant presence and demands, she has nothing to fill up her days. For many persons, boredom is the number one trigger for relapse.

If a large number of your patients are impoverished and have serious deficits in basic life skills (e.g., literacy, or coping skills, such as dealing with job stress and demanding bosses), it is important to get to know the local resources that can help train them in these areas. Recovering people—particularly as they venture out in the world after years of addiction—may be acutely sensitive to rejection, disappointment, and failure. A referral to a training program can improve the chance of finding and keeping a job, and reduce the risk of a patient going back to drinking and drug taking.

Let us look at how we might approach this issue with Alissa.

ALISSA: Yeah, it's true. I am bored. I didn't realize it until Vanessa started school full-time, and I do think I used drugs sometimes because I was bored.

CLINICIAN: Well, that's an important thing to recognize. Because the reasons why you used are often the reasons why you relapse. [Needs assessment]

ALISSA: Yeah, I can see that. But what am I going to do? I haven't had a job for 6 years, and even easy jobs, like working in the fast-food place, are hard to get because there are 10 kids they are going to hire before they even look at me.

CLINICIAN: What about going back to school? [Direct advice]

ALISSA: I don't know. I was never good at school.

CLINICIAN: But I think it could be different now. I can understand your fear that you may not be able to make it in school, but you are more mature and you would know why you were there—it would be your choice, not something your parents made you do. [Empathy]

ALISSA: Hmm, yeah. Well, I often thought that I might like to be an addiction counselor. I see so much pain and suffering for people who suffer from addictions, and I think I can help them.

CLINICIAN: That sounds like a good thing to shoot for. And I happen to know of several training programs here in the city that can help you prepare for school and work. While I was in training for my degree in social work, I interned at a program that sounds perfect for you. They would guide you through the steps you need to take to enter various counseling programs. [Direct advice]

ALISSA: I didn't know there was something like that—I just didn't know where to start.

CLINICIAN: I can get you this information when you are ready.

As you can see, the approach continues to be patient-centered, nondemanding, and informational—helping Alissa think about her plans and not forcing her to make any decisions on the spot.

RELAPSE PREVENTION REVISITED

The next important issue is relapse prevention. Because treatment and support group attendance may be less intense in the later phases of recovery, the important thing is for patients to recognize that they are not "cured," and that they still need to watch out for relapse triggers and uncomfortable situations. Their drinking and drug-taking pattern took years to develop, so changing it is, similarly, a long process.

This does not mean that patients need to dwell constantly on recovery issues; rather, they need to always check themselves and be prepared. The more awareness of potential problems, the more the likelihood that they can be averted.

In practical terms, this means that patients should always consider their motives for being in places where alcohol or drugs will be present, and be careful to leave themselves an "out" in emotional situations that may present triggers. Generally, they should continue to keep an eye on their emotional and physical state to avoid putting themselves in a situation where an impulsive urge becomes a lapse and then a relapse.

Some clinicians claim that relapse is a process and long before the actual drink or drug is taken, patients begin to pull back from recovery. They may start missing counseling or other treatment appointments, avoiding friends in recovery, isolating themselves, or spending more time around old drinking or drug-using friends. They might start to distance themselves from people or return to other behaviors that used to accompany their drinking and drug taking. Counselors often point out these factors as indicators of potential trouble ahead. If you see them, you will want to be sure that your patient is aware of them as well. The problem with the relapse process is that it may be partially unconscious. Awareness can at least give patients a chance to avert it if they were not aware of their direction.

One year after beginning treatment . . .

Bill has now gone 9 months without drinking. His marriage has greatly improved but increasing unhappiness with work has forced him to make some difficult decisions.

Alissa has completed a skills training program and is preparing to enter a community college counseling program. She continues to be drug-free.

Stephen is thinking about marrying his girlfriend but is extremely anxious about whether this is the right decision. He has gone 9 months now without drinking.

Bill has made many changes in his social life, so that it no longer revolves around alcohol. He has become more committed to athletics and spends more time with his wife and children. However, work, which he once found to be his main source of satisfaction, has become more and more unpleasant. He does not want to work 12-hour days anymore and realizes that he is much happier on the racquetball court or playing ball with his kids. He does not see the point in continuing to chase money when he has already achieved his financial goals. He wants to retire, yet having no idea what else to do, he fears that free and unstructured time might cause him to return to drinking.

His story is typical of persons in this phase of recovery. Removing the alcohol has made Bill realize that his career needs to take a backseat, and that to accomplish this, he has to change jobs or careers. If you are not trained in vocational counseling, you should be familiar with career counselors in your area who can help people on all levels of the ladder take on new challenges. There are also numerous books on this topic that may be of use. With a patient like Bill, however, the most important thing you can offer is emotional support. He is adept at research and dealing with the business world, and what he really needs is reassurance that it is OK to slow down and change gears—perhaps do something different. There are probably things he has long dreamed of doing but feels that they would be silly and/or impossible for him. Try to make sure he has support for expressing his ideas and moving toward acting on them.

Alissa, as we can see, has made a big change. She has left her crack cocaine-dealing boyfriend. Her children are doing well in school. Having successfully completed a training program, she has become fully committed to her goal of becoming a counselor; she now spends most her time either attending church, NA, or school. She has filled up the space that alcohol and crack cocaine once occupied in her life. Though she is HIV positive, she has not been sick. Her initial depression and fear that she could do nothing but sit around and wait to die have passed. Discussions with her physician can now safely focus on primary health care issues.

As for Stephen, the changes he wants to make are related to his relationship. Once he stopped drinking, he found he was quite happy on the job and no longer had problems with his boss or lateness. But he has been involved with the same woman on and off throughout his drinking problem and recovery, and while he feels that he loves her, he is not sure he is ready yet to settle down. The dramatic ups and downs of the relationship have served as a distraction once the alcohol was gone, and he wonders if that was his primary reason for sticking with her. He would probably benefit from couple counseling to work this through and determine whether he should marry her.

Relapse prevention tools are usually well established by this point, though the patient should continue self-monitoring for signs of trouble, as necessary. When someone makes any big change, whether it be positive, such as moving to a better job or a better house, or negative, such as breaking off a relationship, there is always an increased risk of relapse, and patients need to remain aware of this.

WHEN TO STOP TREATMENT

The most important question that arises for patients after 6 to 9 months of abstinence is whether to continue treatment or support group attendance. Although 12-step programs recommend lifetime attendance at support groups, many members gradually cut back on the number of meetings they attend after the first year or so. Though some people manage well when they stop going to treatment or support groups, cutting off the support system prematurely can be a major cause of relapse. Because many patients see themselves as "cured" long before they are actually stable in their recovery, it is important to discuss these issues thoroughly.

In many respects, the BRENDA model is a constellation of treatments (e.g., medication, individual counseling, vocational counseling, etc.). One should ask the following questions: What components of treatment stop? What are the signals that a particular component is completed? For example, how long should someone stay on medication? The answer depends on the particular medication and the clinical response of the patient. Some medications, such as methadone, may continue indefinitely. Other medications, such as naltrexone, may be safely discontinued after a sustained period of abstinence.

Since we do not have all the answers for how long one should stay on medication, the safe thing is to continue some counseling or BRENDA visits past the cessation of medication to ensure a proper transition. For example, the use of naltrexone is recommended for 6 to 9 months. Although there are no withdrawal signs associated with discontinuation of naltrexone, patients may feel that the medication has played a major role in their recovery. It is important to support them in their transition off medication. They need to see that they handle unexpected urges and stay abstinent without medication.

Let us look at how you might discuss treatment continuance with Bill. Eight months into treatment, Bill expressed a desire to stop naltrexone.

BILL: Well, I seem to have licked this thing. I haven't touched a drop since my daughter's wedding, and I feel great. Also, my liver enzymes are back to normal ranges. [**B**iopsychosocial evaluation].

CLINICIAN: That sounds good.

BILL: So, do you think I am ready to stop the naltrexone? I don't want to drink. Why should I take the naltrexone anymore? It's also pretty expensive? I mean, I reached my goal, didn't I?

CLINICIAN: Yes, although some ongoing crisis in your life, like your job dissatisfaction, could still throw you off course. What would you think of this? Why don't you go 1 more month on naltrexone, which will give us 6 consecutive months of sustained abstinence? At our next visit, if all seems well, then we'll work out a schedule to discontinue the medication, and some follow-up visits, where we can be sure that you have support following discontinuation of medication should you feel uneasy without the naltrexone. There are no withdrawal signs, but you may feel more temptation to drink, knowing that you aren't taking naltrexone any more. [**D**irect advice]

BILL: OK, I suppose it's better to be safe. We'll go with that plan.

As you can see, this later stage of recovery is about reclaiming one's life. The practitioner's role is much less intensive. You continue with **B**iopsychosocial evaluations to measure progress. For example, periodic blood tests to measure liver enzyme elevations can help confirm that the patient is not drinking. The PSI-32 can be a useful screening tool for emotional distress; a brief overview of how the patient is getting along with employers, friends, and family can give a good estimate of his or her psychosocial status. **R**eporting back to patients on their improvements, not only in their alcohol and other drug use but also in their physical, psychological, and social functioning gives them welcome feedback and can help keep them motivated. Throughout treatment, you remain a consistent source of support and empathy. Patient priority **N**eeds are dynamically changing, so BRENDA visits should continue to assess these needs and goals. In the later stages of recovery, the **D**irect advice is less direct and often geared toward guiding the patients toward their own resources or community referrals. Finally, the patients' responses to treatment recommendations give you feedback on their progress in treatment and help define what is and is not working. It is the **A**ssessment of the patients' responses to treatment recommendations that signals when some components of treatment should end and others should commence.

PART II

The **BRENDA** Approach in Action

■■■■■■

CHAPTER 12

The Case of Bill

A Successful Businessman with Alcohol Addiction

In order to give you a sense of the model in action, the next three chapters each present a full course of BRENDA for the three sample patients we have been following—Bill, Alissa, and Stephen. A typical patient, following detoxification or stabilization, is seen weekly for the first six visits (6 weeks), every other week for the next nine visits (18 weeks), and monthly thereafter for the next 6 months. This covers about 1 full year of treatment. The initial visit is typically for 60–90 minutes, and subsequent sessions last 30–50 minutes. After completion of 1 year of treatment, patients who are stable may be followed every 3 to 6 months for follow-up visits. Patients who are not stable in their recovery after 1 year of treatment are seen more frequently, depending on their progress and clinical status. In the cases that follow, we show how this typical course of visits can vary depending on the patient's needs. In this chapter Bill illustrates treatment for an uncomplicated alcohol addiction. In Chapter 13, Alissa represents a treatment of cocaine and alcohol addiction with severe complications. In Chapter 14, Stephen illustrates how a solid precontemplator can be moved into treatment.

PHASE 1: INITIATING TREATMENT (WEEKS 1–3)

Bill, a 57-year-old male, presents to his medical health care provider for a routine checkup.

Visit 1/Week 1: Focus on Addiction Screening, Biopsychosocial Evaluation, and Patient Safety Needs

Biopsychosocial Evaluation

Biological

Physical exam—liver enlarged
Mild withdrawal symptoms (Alcohol Selective Severity Assessment score of 9)

Psychological

AUDIT—positive for alcohol dependence
PSI-32—indicates little psychological distress (score of 6)

Social

High functioning/high socioeconomic status/high stress
Wife has expressed concern about drinking

Report

The health care provider does not spend a lot of time on presenting the results of the evaluation during this first visit. For example, it is remarked that the liver tenderness can be caused by several factors but the presentation of symptoms is not a cause of immediate concern. Rather, the health care provider suggests that before a clinical diagnosis can be given, more laboratory tests need to be conducted.

Empathetic Understanding

The clinician does not force the issue when Bill says he does not see himself as an alcoholic, nor does he comment about Bill's wife's complaints about his drinking. He collaborates with rather than confronts Bill by offering a chance for more information and a return visit.

Needs Assessment

The heath care provider does not focus on the complete array of patient needs during this visit but focuses on emergent *patient safety needs*. In Bill's case, medical detoxification for alcohol withdrawal is considered but not needed at present.

Direct Advice

Obtain lab tests of liver enzymes.
Return in 1 week to review all the results.

Assessing Response to Direct Advice

While the patient does not believe he has a significant alcohol problem (precontemplative stage), he is willing to have blood tests performed and return in 1 week.

Visit 2/Week 2: Focus on Reporting Results of Biopsychosocial Evaluation and Empathetic Understanding

Biopsychosocial Evaluation

There is no change in Bill's pattern of drinking or relationship with his
   wife.
Bill's liver remains tender.
The lab tests show an elevation in the liver enzymes, most likely due to
   excessive drinking.

Report

The clinician formulates a patient profile based on the results of the Biopsychosocial evaluation. Bill has moderate problems in alcohol, medical, and social areas. He has little or no problem with drugs, employment, emotional distress, or the law. The clinician presents his formulation, focusing on the following facts:

Alcohol dependence is likely:
- Enlarged liver
- Seriously elevated liver enzymes

- Positive AUDIT score for alcohol dependence
- Strained relationship with wife due to her complaining about his drinking behaviors

Empathetic Understanding

The clinician gives Bill time to react and learns the following from Bill's response to the report: Bill remains skeptical that he is an alcoholic, because his concept of an alcoholic is someone who lives in the street and is unable to hold a job. He feels frightened, stunned, and has a sense of shame. The clinician then says why Bill might feel this way: He has treated similar, successful businessmen who felt the same but were able to address the problem successfully.

Needs Assessment

Health safety needs

Alcohol detoxification, possible need for medications to reduce withdrawal symptoms
Alcohol-induced liver disease

Patient priority needs

Primary concern is health
Does not wish to be considered alcoholic
Is not completely opposed to abstinence
May consider improving his relationship with his wife

Direct Advice

Bill is advised to try to reduce drinking on his own.
He is warned to be aware of possible alcohol withdrawal symptoms and to call if they are present.
Naltrexone was mentioned as an option for Bill to consider if he finds it difficult to cut down his drinking this week.
Support groups were discussed but it was agreed not to act on these immediately, because Bill continued to express ambivalence about his need for treatment.
Bill is advised to consider referral to a cognitive-behavioral therapist to learn strategies for coping with craving.

Assessing Response to Direct Advice

Initially reluctant to engage in treatment for alcohol addiction, Bill seems willing to try to cut down on his alcohol drinking for a week. If he is unable to do this on his own, he agrees to try naltrexone and a referral to a therapist. Bill is now in the contemplation stage of treatment. He is not sure if he has a problem, but he is willing to consider the possibility.

Visit 3/Week 3: Focus on Needs and Direct Advice

Biopsychosocial Evaluation

Bill has been unable to abstain from drinking for a week and his craving for alcohol remains high. His mood remains positive and he notes that his wife has been very supportive of his goal to quit drinking.

Report

The clinician reports the facts of Bill's pattern of drinking in the context of Bill's stated desire during the last visit to control his drinking.

Empathetic Understanding

Bill reacts by expressing surprise that he is unable to control his drinking and that his alcohol craving remains high. The clinician empathizes with Bill's experience. Bill says he is now concerned that his drinking is more of a problem than he originally assumed.

Needs

The clinician asks if Bill might need more support than he originally thought. Bill agrees he needs additional support to obtain sobriety and additional strategies to reduce craving and/or cope with craving.

Direct Advice

The health care professional recommends naltrexone, 50 mg per day, and sessions with a cognitive therapist to help Bill learn behavioral strategies to cope with craving. Before prescribing the medication, Bill is given information about naltrexone and discusses with the clinician the importance of taking the medication regularly daily (medication compliance or adherence). Bill says he is not currently taking any pills daily but cannot see why he would have any problem taking the pill right after he eats breakfast every morning. A prescription for naltrexone, 50 mg per day, is written for Bill. In addition, it is suggested that he spend the weekend getting rid of the all the alcohol in his office. This should be accomplished in the presence of someone who knows that he is trying to quit in order to prevent relapse.

Assessing Response to Direct Advice

Bill decides to see a cognitive therapist on a weekly basis for a while in order to change his thinking habits related to drinking. He agrees to start naltrexone and get rid of the alcohol in his office. Bill is now in the action stage of behavioral change.

PHASE 2: EARLY RECOVERY (WEEKS 4–9)

Visit 4/Week 4: Focus on Assessing Patient Response to Direct Advice

Biopsychosocial Evaluation

Since starting naltrexone and addiction counseling, Bill has remained abstinent and his alcohol craving is greatly diminished. He also says he feels more productive. Bill reports no side effects or problems with taking naltrexone.

Report

The clinician gives Bill positive feedback and reviews with him the difference in his ability to abstain this week compared to his inability to abstain the previous week. Also, the dramatic reduction in craving is noted.

Empathetic Understanding

The clinician allows time for Bill to react. Bill feels quite pleased with his progress the past week.

Needs Assessment

The clinician links Bill's improvement to his taking action, and his need for progress in health to his continued sobriety.

Direct Advice

Continue to take naltrexone and attend cognitive therapy visits. Recheck liver enzymes 4 weeks after being on naltrexone.

Assessing Response to Direct Advice

Bill has complied so far with direct advice and appears quite motivated to continue to do so.

Visit 6/Week 6: 6 Weeks in Treatment; Transition to Biweekly Sessions

Biopsychosocial Evaluation/Assessing Direct Advice

Bill reports feeling much better physically, with improved energy and less nagging from his wife. However, he reports that he has not filled the prescription that was written the prior week.

Report

The clinician reviews the results of the repeat liver enzymes test. They are much improved. The clinician also points out how much progress Bill has made since the initial test, although the levels are higher than desirable. The clinician is also pleased that Bill is getting along better with his wife.

Empathetic Understanding

The clinician allows Bill time to react, then asks why he did not fill his prescription. Bill says he stopped the naltrexone because he stopped drinking and feels "cured." Also, he does not like the idea of taking medication—it reminds him that he is ill. The health care professional expresses an understanding of how Bill could feel he no longer needs the medication but reminds him about the results of his Report and that he has only been at this for a little over a month. The health care professional talks to Bill again about the nature of alcohol dependence and how it is a recurrent condition. It is too early to tell if he can maintain long periods of abstinence. Bill says he still feels a desire to drink once in a while.

Needs Assessment

Bill's needs may have changed from a desire for complete abstinence to one of controlled drinking. The clinician asks if Bill's goals have changed. Bill is ambivalent. The health care professional carefully reviews the current goals of treatment and points out that Bill's liver is not completely healed. An occasional drink may lead Bill back to heavy drinking and cause problems in his improving relationship with his wife.

Direct Advice

The health practitioner reviews the benefits of naltrexone and continued sobriety. He advises Bill to remain on naltrexone for at least 6 months. Also, Bill is advised to examine alternative ways to reduce anxiety in social settings where alcohol is being served. Alternative strategies can be developed and practiced in collaboration with the cognitive-behavioral addiction counselor.

Assessing Response to Direct Advice

The clinician asks Bill, "What do you want to do?" Bill agrees to remain on naltrexone and has his prescription filled. He will review with his addiction counselor some techniques to remain abstinent during social situations. Bill has been meeting weekly with the BRENDA clinician through this sixth visit. He is now doing well enough to schedule appointments, starting with the next one, every other week.

Visit 9/Week 12: Focus on Assessing Patient Response to Direct Advice

Biopsychosocial Evaluation

Bill states that he had one drink at his daughter's wedding. He reports that his daughter gave him a disapproving look when she saw him drink, because she was worried that he might get drunk.

Report

After nearly 3 months of continuous sobriety, Bill experienced a slip by having one drink. The health care practitioner points out that this drinking episode differed from his previous drinking pattern, in which he would typically consume six drinks on a drinking occasion. The clinician gives Bill positive feedback on his overall progress, despite the slip.

Empathetic Understanding

The clinician allows Bill to respond. Bill feels guilty for the lapse but was glad that he did not finish the glass and felt no desire to have more. He expressed surprise that he stopped with just one drink and stated that he drank because he did not want people at the wedding to suspect he was an alcoholic.

Needs Assessment

The clinician asks Bill what exactly pushed him to take a drink. Together they work to identify the triggers in the situation and what Bill might need to protect himself. He expresses a need to cope with social pressure without drinking.

Direct Advice

In order for Bill to cope better with social settings where others are drinking, the clinician suggests several strategies, such as using nonalcoholic beverages, avoiding or leaving these high-risk situations, eating something, or using recently acquired cognitive-behavioral skills, to cope with urges to drink.

Assessing Response to Direct Advice

The clinician asks Bill what he thinks of the suggestions. Bill says that he will try to abstain from alcohol in social situations in the future and will discuss the incident further with his cognitive-behavioral therapist. He also says he is glad to be taking naltrexone and attributes his slip of only one drink to the medication.

Visit 10/Week 14: Focus on Assessing Patient Response to Direct Advice

Biopsychosocial Evaluation

Bill discusses how he avoided another potential lapse by arranging ahead of time to have sparkling mineral water served to him at a corporate function. He is finding work very stressful, and feels that although he can still sustain his accustomed level of performance, he does not necessarily wish to do so.

Report

The results of the monthly blood tests show that Bill's liver enzyme results are in the normal range for the first time since beginning treatment.

Empathetic Understanding

The medical health practitioner gives Bill a lot of credit for avoiding the potential lapse and for successfully reducing his liver enzymes. Also, the practitioner offers support to Bill in reassessing his commitment to remain at his current job.

Needs Assessment

Bill remains committed to sobriety and now feels a need to have a job with less stress.

Direct Advice

The clinician discusses possible job changes with Bill but cautions that they are probably better made when he is further along in recovery. Before ending the visit, the clinician reviews all of the treatment options in which Bill is currently involved and confirms that he has continued to see the cognitive therapist and take his naltrexone.

Assessing Response to Direct Advice

Bill remains motivated to take naltrexone and discuss his future career options with his therapist.

PHASE 3: LATER RECOVERY (WEEKS 24–52)

Visit 15/Week 24: 6 Months in Treatment; Transition to Monthly Sessions

*B*iopsychosocial Evaluation

After 3 months of continuous abstinence, Bill is surprised at how much healthier he feels. He has done better in racquetball than he has in years and surprised his son with his agility when they were playing catch. Bill mentions that he has been fighting with his wife some, but he feels that the arguments are at least about real issues, rather than about his drinking, which had caused a great deal of friction before he quit.

*R*eport

The health care professional reviews progress at the 6-month point since treatment began. Since starting to take naltrexone, Bill has only had one slip in alcohol drinking. The liver is no longer tender, and the liver enzymes show that Bill's liver is healing from the damage caused by alcohol. His relationship with his wife has improved; however, now they are talking about "real issues" not related to his alcohol use.

*E*mpathetic Understanding

The clinician gives Bill lots of support about becoming active physically, since exercise can help recovery—both psychologically and physically. Bill feels quite proud of his progress, and the review at 6 months highlights how much progress he has made since beginning treatment.

*N*eeds Assessment

Bill's needs have shifted from controlling his craving and drinking, to dealing with life without alcohol. Also, during the past several sessions, Bill's needs have focused more on his relationship with his wife.

*D*irect Advice

The health care professional discusses with Bill ways he might improve his communication with his wife and encourages continued discussion with his therapist. The clinician mentions couple therapy as an option.

Assessing Response to Direct Advice

Bill sees no need for couple therapy. Before ending the visit, the health care professional reviews all of his current treatment options and confirms that Bill is continuing to see the cognitive therapist and taking his naltrexone.

Visit 17/Week 32

Biopsychosocial Evaluation

A fight with his wife nearly led Bill to a bar, but he thought twice and did not go in.

Report

The clinician had pointed out before Bill began treatment that a situation such as this typically leads to a drinking binge. Yet Bill was able to control the urge for this circumstance. This is significant progress.

Empathetic Understanding

The clinician allows Bill to respond. Then, following Bill's lead, they spend most of the session talking about anger, and how it can be a trigger to relapse. Bill reports disappointment that he still experiences craving for alcohol when he is angry, despite the anger control techniques he learned in cognitive therapy. The medical health care professional points out that it is often difficult to change old habits but despite his temporary desire to drink, Bill was able to resist the impulse. During the session, Bill's affect changes dramatically from anger and disappointment to satisfaction and pride over his ability to resist a drink despite his urge.

Needs Assessment

Bill's most important need is to cope with anger without drinking.

Direct Advice

When asked how he was able to cope with the anger without drinking, Bill reports that he reminded himself that drinking does not solve any problems; then, he spent some time playing racquetball. The health care professional stresses that both are excellent strategies and asks Bill if he can think of other techniques to cope with anger. Bill mentions that he might call a friend, or remember all the wonderful progress he has made.

Assessing Response to Direct Advice

Before ending the visit, the clinician reviews all of Bill's current treatment options. In doing so, the professional finds out that Bill has just discontinued cognitive therapy because he feels he has gotten from it what he wanted. Bill says that this was a mutual decision on his and the therapist's part, and it was a positive parting. The clinician supports him in this decision, but emphasizes how easy it is to return to treatment should the need arise in the future.

Visit 19/Week 40

Biopsychosocial Evaluation

Bill reports continued progress and says he never thought that life without alcohol could be so fulfilling.

Report

The clinician reports that it is now 6 months since Bill's last drink.

Empathetic Understanding

Bill is pleased with his progress in treatment. The health care provider reinforces the fact that Bill has done very well and can feel pride in all the positive changes he has made.

Needs Assessment

Bill has been abstinent for 6 months and now wants to stop the naltrexone.

Direct Advice

The medical practitioner tells Bill that, given his progress in treatment, it is safe to stop taking naltrexone daily. However, if his craving should return, or if he is in a high-risk situation, he may use a naltrexone tablet as needed. Bill is informed that he should immediately report via a phone call if he feels any increased desire to drink, or if he feels less safe without the medication's protection against relapse.

Assessing Response to Direct Advice

Bill agrees to stop taking naltrexone and to report immediately any slips or increase in alcohol craving.

Visit 20/Week 44

Biopsychosocial Evaluation

Bill has successfully stopped the naltrexone. He is pleased with his progress and delighted at how much healthier he feels now that he has quit drinking; he is also much happier in his marriage. His biggest concern now is his growing dissatisfaction with his job. The long hours deprive him of time with his family and friends.

Report

The clinician points out Bill's continued abstinence and improved psychosocial functioning.

Empathetic Understanding

The health care professional points out that, often, people who have a period of sustained sobriety will reassess life goals. It is understandable that the job, with its demanding schedule, was more easily tolerated before Bill discovered the joys of life with his family and friends.

Needs Assessment

Bill now needs most to review occupational options.

Direct Advice

Bill is advised to talk with his boss to see if work conditions can be improved, and to consider talking to his colleagues. The health care professional discusses the possibly of seeing a career counselor to help with his transition and points out that while changing to a less stressful job may lead to extra free time, it could also lead to boredom, which could increase the risk of relapse.

Assessing Response to Direct Advice

Bill decides to take some time off from work and seriously consider finding a new job.

Visit 22/Week 52: Transition from Monthly Treatment Visits to Periodic (Every 3–6 Months) Follow-Up Checks

Biopsychosocial Evaluation

Bill has 9 months of continuous sobriety. It has been 3 months since he stopped taking naltrexone. He reports a full life without alcohol and is increasingly frustrated with his long hours at work. During his vacation from work, he found that he missed his job even less than he imagined, and the free time was filled with pleasant activities with family and friends.

Report

There have been no symptoms of alcohol-related problems for over 6 months, nor is there evidence of liver disease. Bill's relationship with his wife has never been better.

Empathetic Understanding

The clinician congratulates Bill for successfully completing 1 year of treatment and encourages him to explore other vocational options. Bill is reassured that it is OK to pursue activities he has long desired. Bill also expresses concern that with treatment ending, that they will no longer be getting together at monthly intervals. The health care professional reassures Bill that he is available anytime Bill would like to schedule an appointment.

Needs Assessment

Bill needs reassurance that the health care professional remains available should he slip and that it is OK to pursue his dreams.

Direct Advice

Bill is advised to call anytime he needs extra support and that a follow-up visit is scheduled in 3 months. Bill is encouraged to pursue his dreams.

Assessing Response to Direct Advice

Bill agrees to keep in touch.

PHASE 4: FOLLOW-UP VISITS

Follow-Up Visit 4/Status at 2 Years after Initiating BRENDA

Bill retired from his CEO job, though he still acts as a consultant for his company, and has explored setting up a sports program for inner-city children. He is keenly aware that he needs to continue to strike a balance between work and family obligations. Bill continues to be abstinent. He had three more follow-up BRENDA visits after Visit 22 to follow-up his treatment course. At the last visit, his liver enzyme levels were in normal ranges.

SUMMARY

Bill's story of recovery represents a fairly common presentation of someone with an uncomplicated alcohol addiction. The primary challenge in this case was to help him see that he had a problem and to help Bill remain motivated to stay in treatment. It may be difficult to convince someone like Bill, who had not yet suffered terrible consequences from his addiction, that indeed he has a problem that needs to be seriously addressed. The application of the BRENDA method in a primary care setting was ideal, since Bill was more comfortable viewing his problem in medical terms rather than as a "Bowery" type of addiction. The primary care provider skillfully used empathy and pharmacotherapy to help Bill initiate and maintain recovery. The next chapter focuses on the more complicated case of Alissa.

CHAPTER 13

▬

The Case of Alissa

Cocaine and Alcohol Addiction with Severe Psychosocial Complications

Alissa, a 25-year-old woman with three children, presents to a mental health center because she feels depressed and had suicidal thoughts during the week.

PHASE 1: INITIATING TREATMENT (WEEKS 1–4)

Visit 1/Week 1: Focus on Addiction Screening, Biopsychosocial Evaluation, and Patient Safety Needs

Biopsychosocial Evaluation

Biological

Appears malnourished
Jittery, with dilated pupils

Psychological

Suicidal ideation but no definite plans to harm herself
PSI-32—indicates many current symptoms of psychological distress

AUDIT and CAGE (modified to evaluate cocaine use)—positive for both cocaine and alcohol dependence

Social

Social situation problematic—live-in partner is a drug dealer and may be abusive
Unemployed, caring for three small children

Alissa denies recent drug use but admits using crack in the past (several months ago).

Report

The clinician reports to Alissa that her symptoms of malnutrition, anxiety, and emotional distress may be due to drug use.

Empathetic Understanding

The clinician gives Alissa time to react. Alissa is concerned that if she discusses her drug use, she will lose her children. The mental health professional assures Alissa that whatever she says will be held in strict confidence. Alissa expresses shame at her cocaine use, and her therapist expresses support and has a nonjudgmental attitude. Alissa clearly knows she has a problem but is not sure she can do anything about it. She is in the contemplation stage of change.

Needs Assessment

Health safety needs

Reduce feelings of hopelessness and suicidal ideation.
Evaluate physical health for serious medical disorder.

Patient priority needs

Maintain custody of children.
Reduce shame.

Direct Advice

Refer to medical health care provider to evaluate for medical disorders.

Ask if her aunt or another family member can come to next appointment.

Return in 2 days to review treatment options.

Obtain a spot urine drug screen to assess for recent cocaine use.

Assessing Response to Direct Advice

Alissa expresses determination to get help for her multiple problems and agrees to follow through with direct advice.

Visit 2/Week 1: Focus on Direct Advice

Biopsychosocial Evaluation

Biological (results of referral to medical doctor)

Physical exam—recurrent yeast infection, numerous bruises on arms and back.

Urine drug screen—positive for cocaine metabolites.

Psychological

Alissa denies suicidal ideation but complains of low energy, poor concentration, crying spells, poor appetite, and difficulty sleeping.

Social

Alissa reports that her boyfriend hit her several times during the week when she did not have energy to prepare dinner. Her aunt has come with her to the session, as suggested by the therapist the previous week.

Report

Based on the **B**iopsychosocial evaluation, the clinician formulates the following patient profile: cocaine addiction with severe to moderate complications in all seven areas. The mental heath care professional nonjudgmentally reports the facts of the assessment to Alissa. The urine was positive for cocaine, and Alissa herself has reported a lack of control over cocaine use. Her cocaine use is creating financial problems and is also most likely contributing to her emotional problems, such as multiple symptoms of depression.

Empathetic Understanding

Alissa responds with a mix of hopelessness and panic. She feels trapped. The mental health professional expresses understanding for why Alissa feels trapped in her life and offers support and hope. The therapist points to the presence of her aunt at the session as tangible evidence that there are resources to help her in her recovery.

Needs Assessment

Health safety needs

Detoxification of alcohol and cocaine.
Personal safety needs with respect to abusive relationship.
Yeast infection associated with possible sexually transmitted diseases, including HIV infections.
Needs continued monitoring for suicidal ideation and depression.

Patient priority needs

Primary concern is her children.
Requires child care to attend inpatient treatment.

Direct Advice

Participate in inpatient addiction treatment program for 5 days at Center X, if her aunt can take the kids into her home. Alissa has reported that her insurance will only pay for a 1-week inpatient program.
Refer to a psychiatrist to evaluate symptoms of major depression and suicidal ideation for possible antidepressant and naltrexone pharmacotherapy.
Attend support groups. Alissa would greatly benefit from support groups, and they do not cost money or require insurance. She needs a lot of support to achieve abstinence and change her lifestyle, which includes losing her boyfriend. She needs to socialize with healthy, abstinent friends.
Program of twice weekly urine drug screen for cocaine.
Refer for HIV testing.

Assessing Response to Direct Advice

Alissa responds to the advice with determination to address her addiction to cocaine and alcohol. Her aunt volunteers to watch her children while she is away. Alissa will return to continue with care after her discharge from the inpatient program.

Visit 3/Week 4: Focus on Empathetic Understanding

Biopsychosocial Evaluation

It has been over 2 weeks since Alissa's last visit. She states that she has not used cocaine or alcohol during that time. She saw a psychiatrist who prescribed an antidepressant medication. She has not filled her prescription because she says she does not have the money to pay for the pills. She did not show up for her scheduled inpatient admission claiming that she was afraid to leave her kids even though her aunt agreed to watch them. Alissa continues to live with her abusive crack-addicted boyfriend. She has been feeling increasingly despondent and hopeless, and remains ambivalent about treatment. She is still in the contemplation stage. To help move Alissa toward taking action, the therapist will need to be particularly empathetic.

Report

The mental health professional compares her present symptoms with her initial presenting symptoms 4 weeks ago. Except for her report of no cocaine or alcohol use, her physical and emotional health is not improved. Her social situation remains a threat to her physical safety. Finally, the mental health care professional reports that the HIV test came back positive.

Empathetic Understanding

Alissa reports that she feels overwhelmed by all the recommendations that were offered the last session. She does not feel very hopeful about the future and reports that if she had some money, she would consider smoking crack again. Her mental health professional offers support and understanding, and states that it is understandable that

Alissa would feel discouraged and overwhelmed with all that is going on in her life. The therapist suggests that perhaps too many recommendations were offered during the last session and that they should focus on the most pressing problem. In addition, the therapist points out that in addition to the treatment sessions they share, there are other supports available to Alissa. Together they will take each challenge one step at a time and find a way out of this trap. The therapist is using the strategies of building up Alissa's sense of hope, efficacy, and collaboration. This helps to reduce Alissa's fear and her tendency toward denial.

Needs Assessment

While it is imperative that multiple needs be addressed, the therapist focuses on Alissa's feelings of depression and hopelessness, and her lack of helpful social support.

Direct Advice

The therapist provides Alissa with information about the medications and stresses the importance of taking them every day (medication compliance or adherence). With the medications, together with regular attendance in therapy, there is a good chance to improve her symptoms of depression. Once again, the therapist offers Alissa the option of attending an intensive day treatment program or a brief inpatient hospitalization, but Alissa refuses to consider that option. Rather, she asks if she could see the mental health professional several times a week. "I trust you," she says to her mental health professional.

Assessing Response to Direct Advice

Alissa appears much more hopeful and upbeat as the session proceeds. She agrees to take her antidepressant medication and to discuss with her aunt whether she and her kids can move in with her. Finally, she agrees to come in three times per week for individual sessions with the mental heath practitioner. The option of an inpatient referral remains if her clinical situation deteriorates.

PHASE 2: EARLY RECOVERY (WEEKS 5–24)

Visit 6/Week 5

Biopsychosocial Evaluation

Alissa is feeling a little better. She's been taking the medication and attending therapy sessions, but she still seems depressed. Her PSI-32 score has been reduced significantly. The HIV test results show that Alissa has been infected with the HIV virus. Her urine drug screens have been negative for the past 2 weeks.

Report

The therapist reviews the improvement in the PSI-32 scores with Alissa, the negative urine screens for cocaine, and also the results of the HIV test.

Empathetic Understanding

While reviewing the results of the HIV test, Alissa's mood is initially anxious, then increasingly angry. The therapist offers Alissa hope that with aggressive medical treatment, HIV infections can be controlled and she could live a normal life for years to come. Successful examples of people with HIV infections who are living happy, productive lives are presented.

Needs Assessment

Alissa's response to the **R**eport indicates psychological and physical needs related to her HIV status:

Medical treatment for HIV infection
Continued attention to emotional distress, particularly in light of her
   positive HIV status
HIV information and counseling
Continued drug counseling

Direct Advice

The therapist refers Alissa to a physician who specializes in the treatment of HIV infections and offers concrete suggestions for coping with an HIV infection, including behaviors that may put others at risk for becoming infected. Also, the therapist suggests that Alissa attend NA meetings to obtain further social support in her recovery. Attendance at a support group was part of the therapist's initial advice, which seemed overwhelming to Alissa at the time. The therapist mentions it again as an option.

Assessing Response to Direct Advice

Alissa's anger is reduced, yet she remains fearful. She reports that she will make an appointment with the physician as soon as possible and continue with frequent visits with the therapist.

Visit 9/Week 6

Biopsychosocial Evaluation

Alissa continues to show up consistently for the visits with her mental health care professional. She and her children moved into her aunt's place 2 weeks earlier to escape her abusive boyfriend. During the past 2 weeks, her mood has noticeably improved. The urine drug screens remain negative during this time.

Report

The therapist reviews with Alissa her improved mood, drug-free urine tests, and consistent attendance at treatment sessions.

Empathetic Understanding

Alissa feels quite proud of her progress. Her sense of hopelessness has greatly diminished and she feels a special bond with her therapist. Because she feels that she is putting her aunt out by staying with her, she is considering moving back in with her boyfriend. She expresses fear, since her boyfriend has called her; while he claims not to be using crack anymore, she worries that all the triggers of living in the house with him will lead to a relapse. She is also worried that she will be returning to an abusive situation. The therapist recognizes that Alissa has a need not to burden her aunt and to feel that she can manage on her own.

Needs Assessment

Alissa needs to find a safe living environment and, if her only option is to live with her boyfriend, to cope with the reminder cues of using cocaine.

Direct Advice

The therapist suggests that a return to her boyfriend is very likely to risk a return to cocaine use and an abusive situation. Other options are reviewed with Alissa, including the possibility of living in a "safe house" for women recovering from addiction. The therapist states that she will discuss options with a social worker/colleague. For now, it may be best to live with her aunt a few weeks longer.

Assessing Response to Direct Advice

Alissa appears relieved to know that there may be options for her other than to return to her boyfriend's apartment. Before ending the visit, the therapist confirms that she is taking her medication daily and attending NA meetings several times per week. Alissa and the therapist decide to reduce individual sessions to one per week.

Visit 10/Week 7

Biopsychosocial Evaluation

Alissa is having urges to use. Her boyfriend called, and although she did not talk to him, he reminded her of her old life. She is worried about going back home after living with her aunt.

Report

The urine drug screen is negative, and the therapist points out to Alissa that her urine screens have been clean for over a month.

Empathetic Understanding

Alissa feels pride that she did not use but is also scared to realize that "the demon is still lurking." The therapist reinforces the fact that she continues to do remarkably well and states that it is not unusual to experience craving when presented with reminder cues.

Needs Assessment

Alissa needs to cope with her craving for crack cocaine.

Direct Advice

The therapist talks about "people, places, and things" and about "HALT" and discusses ways to deal with living in her old environment, including avoiding unnecessary exposure to high-risk situations. However, it is likely that Alissa will be exposed to cues, so the therapist details specific strategies to reduce craving, such as calling her NA sponsor, letting the wave of craving pass, practicing relaxation responses, and having Alissa remind herself of all the reasons she wants to remain abstinent.

Assessing Response to Direct Advice

Before ending the visit, the therapist confirms that Alissa is taking her medications daily; Alissa is allowed to ask any questions about the medications or report any side effects. She appears determined to maintain her progress and continue with her treatment plan. She also states that she will keep a picture of her three children with her and look at the picture if she experiences cravings for cocaine.

Visit 13/Week 10

Biopsychosocial Evaluation

Alissa forgot to take her medications twice last week. The therapist asks her about it, and she says that she had a cold and also missed an appointment with her psychiatrist. Since she did not eat breakfast, she forgot to take her medications. The therapist asks about her boyfriend, and Alissa says proudly that her NA sponsor helped her get the strength to dump him. The therapist reviews Alissa's cold symptoms and asks about current symptoms.

Report

Alissa is feeling better now than earlier in the week and all her cold symptoms are improved.

Empathetic Understanding

As the therapist discussed Alissa's cold earlier in the week and her missing medications and missed appointment with her psychiatrist, she wonders if there is an important connection. Alissa states that when she felt bad, she began to worry that she was getting sick with AIDS, and her feelings of hopelessness returned. "What's the use taking my meds if I am going to die anyway?" The therapist expresses understanding that it must be tough living with the threat of dying from AIDS. She states that while the possibility of getting AIDS is a real one, Alissa's ability to fight the infection, just like many others who have colds, shows that her immune system is working. The therapist deals with the lapse by not only empathizing with Alissa's fear but also pointing out reasons for hope.

Needs Assessment

Alissa needs to cope with her underlying fear of AIDS and hopeless feelings that her life will be over shortly.

Direct Advice

While the danger of dying from AIDS is possible, it is not likely to happen for some time. On the other hand, missing medications and doctor visits presents an immediate danger to Alissa's recovery. The therapist has Alissa reschedule the psychiatrist visit during the session.

Assessing Response to Direct Advice

Alissa feels relief and a sense of gratitude that the therapist cares enough about her to ensure her commitment to the program of recovery. She agrees to take all the medications as prescribed.

Visit 14/Week 12

Direct Advice and Assessing Response to Direct Advice

Alissa does not show up. The therapist tries calling Alissa at her aunt's, and leaves a message for her to call back. Alissa returns the call but then has to rush. The therapist stresses the importance of Alissa obtaining more medication so she will not run out before the next visit. She agrees to pick up new prescriptions that the therapist asks the psychiatrist to call into the pharmacy that afternoon.

Visit 15/Week 13

Biopsychosocial Evaluation

Alissa apologizes again for missing the appointment 2 weeks ago. She had a beer with her aunt and felt embarrassed because she felt she had blown her whole recovery.

Report

To put this lapse in perspective, the therapist reviews Alissa's progress over the past 3 months: her improvement in mood, her sustained abstinence from cocaine, and her increased self-confidence.

Empathetic Understanding

The therapist talks to Alissa about lapse and relapse, and reassures her that this is OK. She mentions that she continued to take the medications even though she thought she had slipped and was amazed that she did not go on a drinking or cocaine binge. The therapist congratulates her on her progress in treatment.

Needs Assessment

Alissa needs to feel less ashamed about her lapse and to continue attending sessions through difficult times.

Direct Advice

Continue taking medications and make all scheduled sessions.

Assessing Response to Direct Advice

She agrees to not skip appointments if she should have a relapse, but rather to call as soon as possible.

Visit 18/Week 16: Transition to Biweekly Sessions

Biopsychosocial Evaluation

Alissa's mood continues to improve, and she now has 3 months of continuous negative urine screens for cocaine. Her PSI-32 score is in the normal range.

Report

The therapist reviews progress and points out that Alissa has 90 days of continuous abstinence. This is a goal that she thought was impossible when she began treatment. The therapist also reviews the PSI-32 results that have been obtained at monthly intervals. The trend, which has been downward, is now for the first time in the normal range.

Empathetic Understanding

Alissa feel quite proud and begins to talk about other life changes she might want to consider as she continues to recover. She is anxious about doing anything because of her HIV status, but since she has not been really sick, she says she feels that sitting around and waiting to die will not work either. Her aunt has been very generous with letting Alissa stay with her but now Alissa feels like she and her kids are a financial burden.

Needs Assessment

Alissa would like to earn some money to help pay her aunt's expenses She dreams that perhaps someday she could afford her own apartment.

Direct Advice

The therapist asks Alissa to think about what she may want to do as her recovery progresses but tells her to not rush things. The most important priority is to continue to work on her recovery and take care of her children. Before ending the visit, the therapist confirms that Alissa is taking her medications and allows her to ask any questions about the medications or report any side effects.

Assessing Response to Direct Advice

Alissa continues in the maintenance phase of treatment and agrees to attend sessions every other week now.

Visit 20/Week 20

Biopsychosocial Evaluation

While watching a movie in which a young female character was sexually abused, Alissa felt suddenly uncomfortable. She discussed her feelings at an NA meeting and began to remember that her stepdad abused her as a child. She reports feeling increased anxiety and difficulty sleeping. Her urge to use crack has increased during the week.

Report

The therapist reports back that despite this horrible memory and increased urge to use cocaine, Alissa did not use; rather, she looked to support from her NA group.

Empathetic Understanding

Alissa and her therapist discuss the history of sexual abuse. Alissa seems visibly relieved to be able to express her feelings in a supportive environment. She feels fear and rage over what happened to her. The therapist states that Alissa is not alone with these feelings, that, unfortunately, many addicts, particularly females have a history of abuse. Alissa wonders if her past history of abuse helps explain why she put up with her abusive boyfriend for so long.

Needs Assessment

Alissa needs a supportive environment in which to discuss her past history of sexual abuse. She is now in the later stages of recovery, and issues from her past are emerging.

Direct Advice

The therapist invites Alissa to have more frequent sessions to discuss her feelings about her past history of abuse and how it may impact on her life choices now.

Assessing Response to Direct Advice

Alissa says that she is getting enough support from NA to deal with her abuse history. If it becomes a problem, she agrees to see the therapist more frequently.

Visit 22/Week 24

Biopsychosocial Evaluation

Alissa is now well connected in NA. She was able to discuss abuse issues at the NA meetings and was surprised that several fellow members also had similar histories and similar feelings about what happened. She has been drug-free for 5 months and has had only that one lapse with regard to alcohol.

Report

Alissa had given the therapist permission to discuss her progress with her psychiatrist and medical doctor. The therapist reports that the psychiatrist is very pleased about Alissa's compliance with taking the medication and her clinical response. The medical doctor is also pleased that the HIV infection appears to be under good control, with normal levels of immune cells.

Empathetic Understanding

Alissa is pleased with her report but states that she is bored at home since her youngest child has entered kindergarten.

Needs Assessment

Alissa needs to consider vocational goals.

Direct Advice

The therapist discusses possible training and career options.

Assessing Response to Direct Advice

Alissa agrees that if she experiences urges to use cocaine or has a slip, she will inform the therapist. Also, she seems anxious to obtain her general equivalency diploma (GED), since she never completed high school.

PHASE 3: LATER RECOVERY (WEEKS 28–52)

Visit 24/Week 28: Transition to Monthly Sessions

Biopsychosocial Evaluation

Alissa has started a training program so that she can get her GED. She reports feeling very excited about the prospect of getting her degree. She continues to remain free of cocaine use or urges to use.

Report

The therapist reports that it has been 6 months since Alissa last used cocaine.

Empathetic Understanding

Alissa feels quite proud that she has passed another milestone. Despite her initial fear, she is now taking GED classes.

Needs Assessment

Alissa needs to assess career options following completion of her GED.

Direct Advice

The therapist suggests that the urine drug screens are no longer needed and appointments can be decreased to one per month.

Assessing Response to Direct Advice

Alissa agrees that it is no longer necessary to have a program of urine monitoring for drug use and agrees to reduce sessions to one per month.

Visit 26/Week 36

Biopsychosocial Evaluation

Alissa is doing well in her GED program and feels confident that she will pass the test. She continues to attend NA and has reconnected with her church. She sees her ex-boyfriend with another woman in the neighborhood, who has now started using crack cocaine. Rather than being jealous, Alissa is amazed that she feels sorry for her.

Report

Alissa has gone 7 months without any cocaine use.

Empathetic Understanding

Alissa discusses her long-term goal to become a nurse. She likes the idea of helping others. She is having some second thoughts now, since she feels that she would like to help women recover from emotional and sexual abuse. "There is so much suffering. I'd like to be able to help." The therapist supports Alissa in her long-term goals and offers to help obtain information on counseling programs.

Needs Assessment

Alissa continues to assess her long-term career goals.

Direct Advice

The therapist points out that although Alissa is doing remarkably well, it is important to keep the focus on her recovery for now. Some people become complacent when they have over 6 months of clean time. In reviewing how Alissa is doing with her medications, the therapist discovers that she has skipped several doses during the month because "she forgot" and reminds Alissa not to skip any doses, and that if she feels she does not need the meds, to discuss this with her psychiatrist before stopping them.

Assessing Response to Direct Advice

Alissa says she will discuss the need to stay on her antidepressant medication at her next physician visit.

Visit 28/Week 44

Alissa has passed her GED and plans to enroll in a community college counseling program in the spring semester. She is excited at how well she did on the test, and tells the therapist that if she had known it would be that easy, she would not have put it off for all these years.

PHASE 4: FOLLOW-UP VISITS

Status at 1 Year after Initiating BRENDA

Alissa has stayed drug-free for nearly an entire year. Urine and blood tests were repeated at her last visit and all were in normal ranges. She has a new community of friends in NA and at church, and her children are doing well in school. At this time, she is a part-time student in a community college and also has a modest income from watching two of her neighbors' children in the afternoons. She recently discontinued the antidepressant medication and thus far has not had any return of depressive symptoms.

SUMMARY

The challenges in Alissa's case are very different from those in Bill's. Unlike Bill, at the time of beginning treatment, Alissa had moderate to severe problems in a variety of areas of her life, including cocaine and alcohol addiction, severe emotional distress, unemployment, little positive social support, potential legal difficulties over child custody, and a very serious medical illness. Alissa was fortunate to work with a mental health care professional who could address her emotional distress and offered considerable support. Most importantly, the professional offers hope that things will get better. The mental health professional quickly recognized the severity of Alissa's problems and enlisted the support of other health care providers, including an internist who specializes in the treatment of HIV infections, and a psychiatrist who prescribed antidepressant medications. On several occasions, the therapist talked with a colleague/social worker to find options to help Alissa find safe housing and further her education. This is an excellent example of the collaborative approach that the BRENDA method promotes.

CHAPTER 14

The Case of Stephen

A Binge Drinker/Precontemplator

Stephen is a 34-year-old male who has an accident at work. He sees the company nurse, who suspects he was intoxicated.

PHASE 1: INITIATING TREATMENT (WEEKS 1–4)

Visit 1/Week 1: Focus on Biopsychosocial Evaluation

The company nurse conducts biological aspects of the evaluation.

Biopsychosocial Evaluation

Biological

Physical exam—broken leg on the job, alcohol on breath.
Blood tests—slightly elevated liver enzyme levels.

The nurse requires Stephen to see an addiction counselor and arranges the referral.

Visit 2/Week 2: Focus on Biopsychosocial Evaluation and Report

Stephen meets with an addiction counselor as required by the company nurse.

Biopsychosocial Evaluation

Stephen continues to have alcohol binges on weekends. Last weekend, he went to a bar with some friends and had over 10 drinks. He drove home from the bar before he sobered up but arrived safely, without incident.

Psychological

AUDIT—positive for alcohol dependence
PSI-32—indicates few current psychiatric symptoms

Social

Reports alcohol-related absenteeism from work
Believes his job is in jeopardy

Report

Positive Breathalyzer
Somewhat elevated liver enzymes
Positive AUDIT score for alcohol dependence
Has been told by his supervisor that to keep his job he must enter some
     type of rehabilitative program

Conclusion: Alcohol dependence seems likely.

Empathetic Understanding

Stephen does not like the results of the evaluation but is adamant in the claim that he is not an alcoholic. He does not want to be viewed as yet another person who goes to AA meetings and admits to being an alcoholic. He feels that this is too dull a life for him.

Stephen's response indicates that he is a precontemplator and does not believe he has a problem. To help move Stephen into the contemplation stage of change, the counselor needs to provide concrete evi-

dence that Stephen's drinking may be harmful, plus help him recognize
that he is capable of change. The counselor's strategy at this point is to
empathize while further exploring how Stephen feels about the report.
The counselor listens for Stephen's priorities and needs as he defines
them.

Needs Assessment

Primary concern is that he will be asked to give up drinking.
Needs support for a drinking-in-moderation program.
May ultimately require a change in goals to abstinence.
Needs to retain job.

Direct Advice:

The **D**irect Advice formulated by the counselor contains a number of
options from which Stephen can choose. The options are selected in order to accommodate Stephen's health and safety needs as well as his
own main priority of not giving up drinking completely. The counselor
presents the following suggestions as ways that Stephen might be able
to keep his job and not have to give up drinking completely:

Attend or utilize the Internet to be part of Moderation Management
   meetings.
Accurately record drinking pattern and refrain from any binges (five or
   more drinks per drinking occasion).
Attend cognitive therapy, where there is tolerance for the initial goal of
   reducing drinking.
Take naltrexone (along with BRENDA visits) if reducing drinking
   fails.

Assessing Response to Direct Advice

In the precontemplation stage of change, Stephen does not believe he
has a problem.

In order to placate his boss, he is willing to consider a moderation
   drinking program.
He agrees to record his pattern of drinking.

He does not want to consider either cognitive therapy or naltrexone.

Visit 3/Week 3

Biopsychosocial Evaluation

Stephen reports that he drank on Friday, Saturday, and Sunday but each time limited himself to four drinks.

Report

The addiction counselor and Stephen spend some time discussing his broken leg and his three accidents over 2 years. The counselor points out the several incidents of absenteeism at work following a binge the previous day. The facts of Stephen's recent history and assessment provide the concrete evidence that Stephen's drinking may be harmful. Matter-of-factly but consistently keeping the fact before the patient helps him move toward contemplation.

Empathetic Understanding

The counselor reviews with Stephen how he felt about the advice given him last week. He is put off by the thought of giving up his binges. As evidence that he is not an alcoholic, he observes that during the past week he was able to control his drinking. The addiction counselor says that if, indeed, he can control his drinking and not have any binges for at least 1 month, then he may not have a serious drinking problem.

Needs Assessment

Stephen needs to see for himself whether he has a drinking problem.

Direct Advice

The counselor describes some strategies for avoiding binges during this month. Stephen says he does not need any strategies, since he can control his drinking on his own. The counselor states that if Stephen is unable to refrain from binges for even a month, then something should be done to help with a likely drinking problem.

Assessing Response to Direct Advice

Stephen replies that he would be surprised if he cannot avoid a binge for a month and agrees that if he has a binge this month, he will get help for his problem. Stephen moves closer to the contemplation stage.

Visit 4/Week 4

Biopsychosocial Evaluation

Stephen was abstinent all week but then drank heavily over the weekend. He was surprised that he allowed himself to binge drink like that when he wanted to achieve the required abstinence from binges. On Monday, he had a severe hangover and was late for work. His boss warned him that another late day and he would be fired.

Report

The counselor reviews the facts of the initial report and the recent negative consequences Stephen has suffered from drinking.

Empathetic Understanding

The counselor allows time for Stephen to react. Stephen feels disappointed in himself that he could not control his drinking. He finds it difficult to believe he is an alcoholic. The counselor points out that there are many degrees of problem drinking, and some people find it difficult to control their drinking because of the way their bodies react to alcohol. Stephen states that both his father and grandfather were alcoholics. He does not want to be like his father, who could never hang on to a job. The counselor states that, often, the predisposition to drink excessively runs in families, and by addressing the problem now, Stephen can help prevent more severe problems later on.

Needs Assessment

The goal is to reduce shame and start a program to treat Stephen's drinking problem. Stephen would like a program that helps control excessive drinking. He is not ready to give up drinking alcohol entirely.

Direct Advice

The options outlined at Visit 2 are reviewed: Moderation Management meetings, cognitive therapy, and naltrexone.

Assessing Response to Direct Advice

Stephen agrees to try the Moderation Management program. As provided in the program, he will attempt to remain completely abstinent for several weeks before he tries controlled drinking.

PHASE 2: EARLY RECOVERY (WEEKS 5–24)

Visit 5/Week 5

Biopsychosocial Evaluation

Stephen does not drink over the weekend and now has about 7 days of continuous abstinence. A huge fight with his girlfriend almost resulted in a relapse, but he was able to stop himself.

Report

This is the first week with no drinking in years for Stephen.

Empathetic Understanding

Stephen feels quite proud of his progress but is surprised how his craving increased after the fight with his girlfriend.

Needs Assessment

Stephen needs to control his urges.

Direct Advice

The addiction counselor discusses triggers for relapse, such as HALT, and how to avoid them. In addition to his Internet program to learn to moderate his drinking, the counselor suggests that Stephen check out support groups in person.

Assessing Response to Direct Advice

Stephen agrees to try to avoid triggers for his drinking and will look for support groups in his community.

Visit 6/Week 6

Biopsychosocial Evaluation

Stephen says he was abstinent most of the time during the last week but then mentions that he missed another day of work due to a hangover. Fortunately, the supervisor was out that day and there were no consequences for missing work.

Report

After a week of complete abstinence, Stephen has jeopardized his job because of another binge. The counselor reviews with Stephen his pattern of drinking over the past 6 weeks. Despite many days without any alcohol, nearly every time Stephen has a drink, he binges. The counselor again presents nonjudgmentally the facts of Stephen's drinking and its negative consequences.

Empathetic Understanding

Stephen feels worried about his drinking: "How can I be so stupid?" The counselor responds that it is not stupidity that causes Stephen to drink and offers support, telling Stephen that there are ways to help him with his problem. Empathy can deepen Stephen's awareness of the problem, but he also needs reinforcement to know that change is possible.

Needs Assessment

Stephen needs more strategies to help reduce excessive drinking.

Direct Advice

The counselor suggests that Stephen try a period of complete abstinence and also start taking naltrexone, a medication that can help control urges and reduce binges. Information on naltrexone is presented, together with how this medication may help Stephen obtain the abstinence he is trying to achieve on his own.

Assessing Response to Direct Advice

Stephen is pessimistic that he can remain abstinent but agrees to see the physician for a naltrexone prescription. He appears ambivalent about trying the medication.

Visit 8/Week 8: Transition to Biweekly Sessions

Biopsychosocial Evaluation

Stephen reports that he has not drunk for 2 weeks and states that he has had little craving for alcohol since he began the naltrexone 10 days ago.

Report

The counselor reports that 2 weeks is Stephen's longest period of sobriety since starting treatment and that the reduction in craving coincides with his starting the medication.

Empathetic Understanding

Stephen feels very satisfied with his progress over the past 2 weeks and is more hopeful that he can abstain from drinking.

Needs Assessment

Continued abstinence or, at the very least, an absence of episodes of binge drinking.
Continued motivation to remain on the medication and attend treatment sessions.

Direct Advice

The counselor points out that Stephen was initially ambivalent about taking the medicine and reminds him about his need to stop drinking. Now, since he has been active in treatment and compliant with taking the medication, there are clear reductions in drinking and urges. Stephen is encouraged to keep taking his medications and attending treatment sessions. At Stephen's request, sessions are reduced to one every other week. Before ending the visit, the counselor confirms that Stephen is taking naltrexone daily and encourages him to ask any questions about the medication or report any side effects.

Assessing Response to Direct Advice

Stephen is pleased with his progress and with the recommended reduction in frequency of visits. He agrees to take the naltrexone as prescribed.

Visit 9/Week 10

Biopsychosocial Evaluation

Stephen reports that he has not been drinking for a month, and that he would like to start the program of moderate drinking.

Report

The counselor reviews Stephen's progress during the past weeks. Not only has Stephen not been drinking but also his work performance has improved and there have been no arguments with his girlfriend.

Empathetic Understanding

The counselor wonders why Stephen wants so badly to drink occasionally, since the past month without any drinking has not been so difficult and has led to improved performance at work, and possibly improved relations with his girlfriend. Stephen states that he is not an alcoholic (like his father) and there may be times when he would like to share a drink with some friends. The counselor reports that he understands why Stephen would not want to be compared to his father or be different from his friends at social functions.

Needs Assessment

While the counselor feels that complete abstinence is the best option for Stephen, he begins to understand Stephen's desire to feel that he is not like his father and to feel accepted by his peers.

Direct Advice

The counselor states concern about a program of moderate drinking given Stephen's drinking pattern before beginning treatment, and the risk that drinking could lead to a loss of his job. Rather, the counselor recommends a program in which abstinence is the goal. Before ending the visit, the counselor confirms that Stephen is taking naltrexone daily and asks if Stephen has any questions about the medication or wants to report any side effects.

Assessing Response to Direct Advice

Stephen states that he believes he can learn to drink moderately but agrees to consider a goal of abstinence if he has binges.

Visit 10/Week 12

Biopsychosocial Evaluation

Stephen is struggling after 2 weeks of attempting moderation. He does fine during the week for the most part but spends a great deal of time thinking about drinking and wishing he could have more alcohol than he is supposed to have. On weekends, particularly if he is fighting with his girlfriend, he exceeds his limits and becomes very drunk. The counselor finds out (only by asking) that Stephen has not been taking his naltrexone regularly. Stephen says he does not always think he needs it, and by the time he realizes he is drunk, he does not feel right about swallowing pills. Because of the past weekend binge, he was late for work on Monday. His employer is "on to" this pattern of coming to work late on Monday and warned Stephen that he must be in treatment for his alcohol problem to continue his employment.

Report

The counselor reviews Stephen's pattern of drinking and the consequences of his continued binges.

Empathetic Understanding

Stephen feels upset with himself and discouraged. The counselor offers support and hope that this pattern can change.

Needs Assessment

Stephen feels he needs to do something drastic about his drinking and would like to consider a goal of abstinence.

Direct Advice

The counselor provides Stephen with more education on how naltrexone works and discusses strategies for ensuring that Stephen takes the medication over the weekend. In addition, the counselor suggests weekly sessions to learn skills for coping with craving. Finally, he suggests that Stephen attend AA or Rational Recovery meetings.

Assessing Response to Direct Advice

Stephen agrees both to see the counselor weekly for a few visits and to try one AA meeting per week.

Visit 14/Week 16

Biopsychosocial Evaluation

Stephen has been abstinent for the past four BRENDA visits (for the last month). However, he nearly slipped because he chose not to take the naltrexone on a day when he was going to a bar to meet a friend.

Report

The counselor reports that there has been significant progress since Stephen has been consistently attending BRENDA sessions and taking his medication. Also, he points out that Stephen's failure to take his naltrexone can herald a desire to drink.

Empathetic Understanding

Until the counselor discussed the situation, Stephen did not recognize that he could be setting himself up for a slip. His feelings about being on naltrexone are explored. Stephen states that while he would rather control his drinking on his own, he now feels comfortable being on the medication.

Needs Assessment

Stephen needs to continue to avoid high-risk situations and learn ways to cope with craving, and to avoid slips and binges.

Direct Advice

Stephen is advised to take the medication and agrees to watch his thought processes more carefully to avoid these types of situations.

Assessing Response to Direct Advice

Stephen agrees to keep track of situations that elicit craving.

Visit 18/Week 24: Transition to Monthly Sessions

Biopsychosocial Evaluation

It has been about 3 months since Stephen's last drink. He is amazed that he has fewer urges to drink and surprised to report that fights with his girlfriend have not escalated the way they did in the past.

Report

The counselor points out Stephen's progress during the past 6 months since treatment began, especially in the past 3 months. Progress is related to consistent attendance at treatment sessions and adherence to taking his medication.

Empathetic Understanding

Stephen is quite pleased with his progress. The counselor reinforces Stephen's progress during treatment.

Needs Assessment

Stephen desperately wants to hear a friend's band play at a bar and feels ready to deal with the situation. He has not had a drink for 3 months now and feels that his drinking problem is behind him.

Direct Advice

The counselor reviews the strategies for coping with urges and role-plays how Stephen may refuse a drink if it is offered. Before ending the visit, the counselor confirms that Stephen is taking naltrexone daily and asks him about any side effects. The counselor and Stephen agree to reduce the sessions to 1 per month.

Assessing Response to Direct Advice

Stephen expresses a desire to remain sober and feels confident that he can go into a bar to hear his friend without drinking. He feels connected to his support group in AA and attends weekly meetings.

PHASE 3: LATER RECOVERY (WEEKS 25–52)

Visit 20/Week 32

Biopsychosocial Evaluation

Stephen is still attending AA. He recently was given a raise at work "because he has been so committed to the job." Surprised at how supportive his girlfriend is being, he feels like he is really starting to have a serious relationship for the first time in his life.

Report

It is now 4 months since Stephen last drank. He continues to show improvement in his vocational and social functioning.

Empathetic Understanding

Stephen is feeling anxious about the possibility of making a long-term commitment to his girlfriend. He wonders out loud if he should settle down at this time of his life. The counselor offers support and gives Stephen the opportunity to express his fears and concerns.

Needs Assessment

Stephen remains committed to sobriety but wonders about his long-term goals with respect to his girlfriend.

Direct Advice

The counselor discusses ways of coping with strong emotions without using alcohol to numb the feelings. Before ending the visit, the counselor confirms that Stephen is taking naltrexone daily and has no significant side effects.

Assessing Response to Direct Advice

Stephen decides he does not have to make a decision on this matter right away and feels relieved. He wonders if he has a lifelong pattern of avoiding commitment.

Visit 22/Week 40

Biopsychosocial Evaluation

It is now 6 months since Stephen's last drink.

Report

The counselor reviews progress during the preceding month and relates it to continued motivation to attend treatment sessions and support groups, and to maintain medication adherence.

Empathetic Understanding

Stephen feels quite proud of his progress. The counselor reinforces the fact that Stephen is doing well.

Needs Assessment

Stephen wants to discontinue the naltrexone. Although it has been helpful, Stephen believes it is no longer necessary.

Direct Advice

Since Stephen has completed 6 months without drinking, the counselor suggests that he talk with the physician who prescribed the naltrexone. From the counselor's perspective, it is very reasonable to see how Stephen does off naltrexone, with the option of going back on the medicine if there is a return of drinking.

Assessing Response to Direct Advice

Stephen agrees to discuss stopping naltrexone with his physician. Meanwhile, he will continue to use coping strategies to deal with craving and continue to attend weekly AA meetings.

Visit 25/Week 52

Biopsychosocial Evaluation

Stephen successfully discontinued the naltrexone and considers proposing to his girlfriend.

Report

The counselor points out that Stephen has about 9 months of continuous sobriety and there are important improvements in his social relationships.

Empathetic Understanding

Stephen is terrified but feels that he will lose his girlfriend if they do not go forward soon. The counselor discusses the relationship and how it was linked with Stephen's drinking and recovery, and what it means to him.

Needs Assessment

Stephen needs to understand his ambivalent feelings about committing to his girlfriend.

Direct Advice

The counselor suggests the possibility of couple counseling with a specially trained couple therapist. The counselor recommends follow-up visits at 3-month intervals to monitor further Stephen's drinking status.

Assessing Response to Direct Advice

Stephen agrees to consider couple counseling and will talk it over with his girlfriend. Meanwhile, he is pleased with his course of treatment and agrees to regular follow-up visits. He will also continue to attend AA meetings.

PHASE 4: FOLLOW-UP VISITS

Status at 2 Years after Initiating BRENDA

Stephen has been alcohol-free for 21 months and believes he will not go back to drinking given all the good things that have happened to him since he chose abstinence. His job is steady, and he has not taken any sick time for over a year. He married his girlfriend 3 months ago and is now a supervisor at work.

SUMMARY

In Stephen's case, the major challenge for the addiction counselor was to help Stephen recognize that he had a problem and to find a treatment that best served his needs. Initially, Stephen claimed quite adamantly that he did not have a problem. Unlike Alissa, who recognized the severity of her problem but tried to hide her addiction because of possible legal sanctions, Stephen could see no reason why he could not continue to drink. Like Bill, Stephen did not recognize his addiction to alcohol, but at least Bill saw that drinking alcohol presented a health problem.

The addiction counselor skillfully avoided direct confrontation and managed to keep Stephen engaged in treatment. After unsuccessful attempts to control his drinking, Stephen gradually came to see that he had an alcohol addiction and was at that point open to the use of medications and the support of AA. The counselor's patience eventually paid off, as Stephen remained motivated in treatment. The addiction counselor using the BRENDA method, in collaboration with a physician who prescribed naltrexone, helped Stephen successfully achieve a stable period of abstinence.

Instruments

CAGE QUESTIONNAIRE

C   Have you ever felt the need to **C**ut down on your drinking? [drug use]

A   Have you ever felt **A**nnoyed by someone criticizing your drinking? [drug taking]

G   Have you ever felt bad or **G**uilty about your drinking? [drug use]

E   Have you ever had a drink first thing in the morning to steady your nerves and get rid of a hangover (**E**ye-opener)? [or a drug to take away withdrawal symptoms or drug craving]

Adapted from Mayfield, McLeod, et al. (1974). Copyright 1974 by the American Psychiatric Association. Adapted by permission.

ALCOHOL USE DISORDERS IDENTIFICATION TEST (AUDIT)

AUDIT is a brief structured interview developed by the World Health Organization that can be incorporated into a medical history. It contains questions about recent alcohol consumption, dependence symptoms, and alcohol-related problems.

Begin the AUDIT by saying, "Now I am going to ask you some questions about your use of alcoholic beverages during the past year." Explain what is meant by alcoholic beverages (e.g., beer, wine, liquor [vodka, whisky, brandy, etc.]). Record the score for each question in the area on the right side of the question.

How often do you have a drink containing alcohol?

Never	(0)
Monthly or less	(1)
2 to 3 times a month	(2)
2 to 3 times a week	(3)
4 or more times a week	(4)

How many alcoholic drinks do you have on a typical drinking day?

None	(0)
1 or 2	(1)
3 or 4	(2)
5 or 6	(3)
7 or 9	(4)
10 or more	(5)

How often do you have six or more drinks on one occasion?

Never	(0)
Less than monthly	(1)
Monthly	(2)
Weekly	(3)
Daily or almost daily	(4)

Adapted from Babor, de la Fuente, Saunders, and Grant (1992). Copyright 1992 by World Health Organization. Adapted by permission.

How often during the last year have you found that you were unable to stop drinking once you had started?

Never	(0)
Less than monthly	(1)
Monthly	(2)
Weekly	(3)
Daily or almost daily	(4)

How often during the last year have you failed to do what was normally expected of you because of drinking?

Never	(0)
Less than monthly	(1)
Monthly	(2)
Weekly	(3)
Daily or almost daily	(4)

How often during the last year have you needed a drink first thing in the morning to get yourself going after a heavy drinking session?

Never	(0)
Less than monthly	(1)
Monthly	(2)
Weekly	(3)
Daily or almost daily	(4)

How often during the last year have you had a feeling of guilt or remorse after drinking?

Never	(0)
Less than monthly	(1)
Monthly	(2)
Weekly	(3)
Daily or almost daily	(4)
Never	

How often during the last year have you been unable to remember what happened the night before because you were drinking?

Never	(0)
Less than monthly	(1)
Monthly	(2)
Weekly	(3)
Daily or almost daily	(4)

Have you or someone else been injured as a result of your drinking?

Never	(0)
Less than monthly	(1)
Monthly	(2)
Weekly	(3)
Daily or almost daily	(4)

Has a relative, friend, or a doctor or other health worker been concerned about your drinking or suggested you cut down?

Never	(0)
Less than monthly	(1)
Monthly	(2)
Weekly	(3)
Daily or almost daily	(4)

Record the total specific items. A score of 8 is the cutoff point for a positive test.

SUBSTANCE USE DISORDERS SCREEN

How often do you take recreational drugs?

Never	(0)
Monthly or less	(1)
2 to 3 times a month	(2)
2 to 3 times a week	(3)
4 or more times a week	(4)

How often do you take enough drugs that your functioning is at least moderately impaired?

Never	(0)
Less than monthly	(1)
Monthly	(2)
Weekly	(3)
Daily or almost daily	(4)

How often during the last year have you found that you were unable to stop taking drugs once you had started?

Never	(0)
Less than monthly	(1)
Monthly	(2)
Weekly	(3)
Daily or almost daily	(4)

How often during the last year have you failed to do what was normally expected of you because of drug use?

Never	(0)
Less than monthly	(1)
Monthly	(2)
Weekly	(3)
Daily or almost daily	(4)

How often during the last year have you needed drugs as soon as you awaken to get yourself going or to avoid withdrawal symptoms?

Never	(0)
Less than monthly	(1)

Adapted by the first author from the AUDIT without endorsement by the World Health Organization.

Monthly	(2)
Weekly	(3)
Daily or almost daily	(4)

How often during the last year have you had a feeling of guilt or remorse after taking drugs?

Never	(0)
Less than monthly	(1)
Monthly	(2)
Weekly	(3)
Daily or almost daily	(4)

How often during the last year did you experience serious physical symptoms related to your drug use (i.e., for heroin, withdrawal or overdose; for cocaine, overdose, more than 24 hours awake, paranoia, or seriously elevated heart rate; for marijuana, oversleeping or forgetfulness; for multiple drugs, overdose or any of above symptoms)

Never	(0)
Less than monthly	(1)
Monthly	(2)
Weekly	(3)
Daily or almost daily	(4)

Have you or someone else been injured as a result of your drug use?

Never	(0)
Less than monthly	(1)
Monthly	(2)
Weekly	(3)
Daily or almost daily	(4)

Has a relative, friend, or a doctor or other health worker been concerned about your drug use or suggested you cut down?

Never	(0)
Less than monthly	(1)
Monthly	(2)
Weekly	(3)
Daily or almost daily	(4)

Record the total specific items. If you score higher than 7, you should get a further evaluation because you may have a substance problem.

PSYCHOLOGICAL SYMPTOM INVENTORY—32 (PSI-32)

Below is a list of problems and complaints that people sometimes have. Please read each one carefully and circle the number that best describes how much you were bothered by that problem during the past week. PLEASE CHOOSE ONLY ONE. For the past week, how much were you bothered by:

	Not at all	A little bit	Moderately	Quite a bit	Extremely
1. Nervousness or shakiness inside	0	1	2	3	4
2. Unwanted thoughts, words, or ideas that won't leave your mind	0	1	2	3	4
3. Loss of sexual interest or pleasure	0	1	2	3	4
4. Trouble remembering things	0	1	2	3	4
5. Worried about sloppiness or carelessness	0	1	2	3	4
6. Feeling easily annoyed or irritated	0	1	2	3	4
7. Feeling low in energy or slowed down	0	1	2	3	4
8. Thoughts of ending your life	0	1	2	3	4
9. Crying easily	0	1	2	3	4
10. Feeling shy or uneasy with the opposite sex	0	1	2	3	4
11. Feeling of being trapped or caught	0	1	2	3	4
12. Suddenly scared for no reason	0	1	2	3	4
13. Blaming yourself for things	0	1	2	3	4
14. Feeling blocked in getting things done	0	1	2	3	4
15. Feeling lonely	0	1	2	3	4
16. Feeling blue	0	1	2	3	4
17. Worrying too much about things	0	1	2	3	4
18. Feeling no interest in things	0	1	2	3	4
19. Feeling fearful	0	1	2	3	4
20. Your feelings being easily hurt	0	1	2	3	4
21. Feeling others do not understand you or are unsympathetic	0	1	2	3	4
22. Feeling that people are unfriendly or dislike you	0	1	2	3	4

Adapted by the author from Derogatis, Lipman, et al. (1973).

23. Having to do things very slowly to insure correctness	0	1	2	3	4
24. Feeling inferior to others	0	1	2	3	4
25. Trouble falling asleep	0	1	2	3	4
26. Having to check and double-check what you do	0	1	2	3	4
27. Difficulty making decisions	0	1	2	3	4
28. Having to avoid certain things, places, or activities because they frighten you	0	1	2	3	4
29. Your mind going blank	0	1	2	3	4
30. Feeling hopeless about the future	0	1	2	3	4
31. Trouble concentrating	0	1	2	3	4
32. Feeling tense or keyed up	0	1	2	3	4

APPENDIX B

Naltrexone Pharmacotherapy for Alcohol Dependence

This appendix reviews information on naltrexone and specific prescribing practices. Naltrexone has been studied as a treatment in research for more than two decades and has been approved for the treatment of opiate addiction for over 12 years. In 1994, the U.S. Food and Drug Administration approved it specifically for the treatment of alcohol dependence.

For additional information on the risk and benefits of naltrexone, see a review by Berg, Pettinati, et al. (1996).

DOSAGE AND ADMINISTRATION

The standard dose for naltrexone treatment of alcohol dependence is 50–100 milligrams/day taken orally once daily. Naltrexone should be taken with food in order to minimize gastrointestinal side effects. If side effects occur, changing the time of taking the medication can often eliminate them (e.g., from morning dosing to evening or nighttime dosing, or split the dose so that half is taken in the morning and half in the evening).

There are no data on how long naltrexone pharmacotherapy should be given. A typical course of suggested treatment is 6 months. It is also recommended that naltrexone pharmacotherapy be given in conjunction with a behavioral treatment to assist in ensuring good adherence to taking the medication, educating the patient about alcohol dependence and treatments, and, in general, helping the patient maintain abstinence and a healthy lifestyle. Also, naltrexone pharmacotherapy is compatible with attending support groups in the community.

As mentioned earlier, for safety purposes, liver enzyme tests should be run prior to initiation of treatment and monthly throughout the course of treatment. Monitoring side effects and discussing medication-taking strategies should also be done at each visit.

Experience with overdose of naltrexone in humans is limited. Patients who have overdosed should be treated symptomatically in an inpatient setting.

There is little known at the time of this writing on the safety of combining naltrexone with antidepressants. The few case reports published today report the combination is well tolerated.

PHARMACOKINETICS/MECHANISM OF ACTION

Naltrexone is a competitive opiate antagonist, with specific action at opiate receptor subtype 5, kappa. It is nearly a pure antagonist—while it may have some agonist properties, they pale in contrast to its potent antagonist action. Naltrexone is 17 times more potent than nalorphine and twice as potent as naloxone.

Naltrexone's opiate blocking action can persist up to 72 hours. After oral administration, absorption is rapid and almost complete (approximately 96%). However, only 5–20% of the medication reaches systemic circulation unchanged, due to extensive first-pass metabolism in the liver. Protein binding is between 21% and 28%. Naltrexone is widely distributed throughout the body, and antagonist activity seems to be related to plasma and tissue concentrations. Cerebrospinal fluid concentrations are presently not known.

The primary metabolite of naltrexone is 6-beta-naltrexol, which has some antagonist action but is less potent. Chronic administration does not appear to cause an accumulation of either naltrexone or 6-beta-naltrexol.

Both naltrexone and its metabolites conjugate with glucaronic acid after metabolism in the liver. Both drug and metabolite may undergo enterohepatic recirculation. Only 2% of the drug is excreted unchanged in urine within 24 hours.

Elimination half-life of naltrexone ranges from 4 to 10 hours, but a terminal elimination half-life of 96 hours has also been reported. For 6-beta-naltrexol, the elimination half-life is roughly 14 hours.

DRUG INTERACTION PRECAUTIONS

Because naltrexone blocks the action of opiate painkillers, these are contraindicated, since they are made ineffective or less effective by naltrexone's primary action. Patients undergoing any kind of surgery that will require the use of opiate painkillers should discontinue naltrexone at least 72 hours before preoperative medications are initiated.

In case of accident or emergency, naltrexone patients should carry a card stating that they are on naltrexone to inform medical personnel that alternate methods of pain management or higher doses of opiate drugs may be needed. Naltrexone may not completely antagonize the respiratory depression caused by extremely high opiate doses; so appropriate precautions should be taken.

Warning for patients on antipsychotics: Naltrexone can cause an increase in somnolence and lethargy in patients who are simultaneously receiving phenothiazines.

SIDE EFFECTS

The data from the largest study of naltrexone treatment for alcohol dependence found that the most common side effect was nausea, which occurred in 10% of patients, while 3% actually vomited. Other side effects were headache (7%), dizziness (4%), fatigue (4%), insomnia (3%), anxiety (2%), depression (5-7%), suicidal ideation (2%), and sleepiness (2%).

In alcohol studies, side effects were severe enough to warrant discontinuation in 5–10% of patients. For most patients, however, side effects are mild or only present for a short period after initiation of treatment.

CONTRAINDICATIONS

Naltrexone should not be prescribed for people with severe liver or kidney damage, pregnant women, or patients who cannot achieve abstinence for at least 5 days prior to the start of the pharmacotherapy. It is also contraindicated for patients with a known sensitivity to naloxone or nalmefene, which are structurally similar compounds.

In opiate dependence, naltrexone can precipitate withdrawal if patients are not opiate-free for at least 7 days prior to initiating naltrexone, although there are some detoxification techniques currently under investigation that can shorten this time period.

Patients with chronic pain requiring opiate treatment also cannot take naltrexone, as it will prevent their painkillers from being effective.

In rare instances, naltrexone has been known to cause hepatoxicity, though most alcohol-dependent patients with elevated liver enzymes at treatment entry show an improvement in liver function with naltrexone due to a decrease in alcohol intake. However, for safety purposes, liver enzyme tests should be run prior to initiation of treatment and monthly throughout the course of treatment.

PATIENTS' FREQUENTLY ASKED QUESTIONS ABOUT NALTREXONE

What is naltrexone?

Naltrexone is a nonaddictive medication that blocks opiate receptors in the brain. In this way, opiates such as heroin are blocked in their ability to produce a drug high. More recently, studies have shown that naltrexone also blocks the craving for alcohol and the high associated with drinking. For many people who find that they have difficulty controlling their alcohol use once they start drinking, naltrexone reduces the craving in which one drink leads to another. When combined with the help of psychosocial support system, naltrexone can dramatically reduce the chance of a relapse to alcohol drinking.

What are the side effects of naltrexone?

Most people do not report side effects when they take naltrexone. However, in cases when side effects have been reported, they are reportedly mild in nature and gradually disappear after a few days. Side effects of naltrexone include nausea, irritability, fatigue, and dizziness. When people report side effects, it has been found that reducing the amount of naltrexone, taking it with food, or taking it before bedtime greatly reduces, or diminishes, these complaints. If however, you still experience discomfort after implementing these strategies, you should contact your doctor for further assistance.

Is naltrexone safe to use?

Naltrexone is an FDA-approved drug that has been on the market since 1985 for the treatment of opiate addiction, and since 1994 for the treatment of alcoholism. Naltrexone has also been approved in over a dozen other countries and is prescribed to thousands of people each year, throughout the world. Studies show that in typical doses used to treat alcoholism, naltrexone is very safe. However, it should not be taken if you use narcotics on a regular basis. Likewise, if you currently suffer from severe liver damage, you should consult with your doctor as to whether you are a good candidate for taking naltrexone.

Should I take naltrexone?

If you are having trouble controlling your drinking, then you should consider taking naltrexone. Naltrexone is safe and effective in the treatment of alcoholism. Naltrexone is not a crutch or a cure-all, but it makes it much easier for people to stop using alcohol.

How long should I take it?

There is no defined time frame that people are assigned when taking naltrexone. However, it is suggested that for optimum results you should have a minimum of 6 months of complete sobriety before you stop taking the medication. It is not uncommon for people to stay on it for a year or more, and some people stay on naltrexone for years, or use naltrexone when they experience craving or are in a situation where alcohol craving is likely to increase.

Can I take naltrexone if I am on other medications?

It is safe to take naltrexone with other medications, unless you are taking opiate-containing medications such as codeine, Percocet (oxycodone and acetaminophen), Demerol (meperidine hydrochloride), and especially methadone. If you have been on opiate pain killers for more then a few days, the use of naltrexone can produce severe withdrawal symptoms from these medications. Naltrexone has been safely used in combination with selective serotonin reuptake inhibitors (SSRIs) and other antidepressants such as Prozac (fluoxetine), mood stabilizers such as lithium, anxiety-reducing medications such as Xanax (alprazolam) or Valium (diazepam), blood pressure medications, and non-narcotic pain relievers such as aspirin or Tylenol (acetaminophen). Please consult with your doctor when combining naltrexone with other medications.

What will happen if I take an opiate medication while taking naltrexone?

Patients who take opiates in small dosages will not experience the drug's effects due to the blocking of the opiate receptors in the brain. However, large doses of narcotics will override naltrexone's blocking effect. If you are addicted to opiates or have been taking opiates such as methadone chronically, naltrexone can bring on a severe withdrawal reaction. If you discontinue naltrexone because you are taking an opiate-based drug, it is important to contact your doctor before starting naltrexone again.

Can I take naltrexone if I am pregnant or nursing?

Studies have not yet been performed reporting the possible risks associated with naltrexone and pregnancy. It is also unknown whether naltrexone can be transmitted through breast milk. Like all medications used during pregnancy, one must weigh the risks and benefits. The effects of alcohol on the fetus are well documented, however, so above all, do not drink during pregnancy.

What if I drink alcohol while on naltrexone?

Naltrexone is found to block the "high" associated with alcohol intake. Therefore, many people report not wanting to drink as much. However, if you do
drink alcohol while you are taking naltrexone, you will not become sick.

*What if I get in an accident and need opiate pain relievers while taking
naltrexone?*

Many people carry a medical alert card with them at all times, stating that they
are on naltrexone, because in case of an accident, it will take higher doses of
opiate pain relievers to reduce their pain. It is possible to override the effects of
naltrexone with higher dosages of opiates or to be prescribed a comparable
medication that is not an opiate.

Will I become addicted to naltrexone?

Naltrexone does not have addictive properties. Therefore, it is perfectly safe to
take naltrexone for an extended amount of time without worrying about withdrawal symptoms.

If I take naltrexone, do I need additional treatment?

For optimal results, it is suggested that naltrexone be used in combination with
psychosocial support. Research finds that sobriety is obtained and maintained
when naltrexone is used as part of an overall treatment plan. Each individual
however, can choose the plan that works best for him or her.

In rare instances, naltrexone has been known to cause hepatotoxicity,
though most alcohol-dependent patients with elevated liver enzymes at treatment entry show an improvement in liver function with naltrexone due to a decrease in alcohol intake. However, for safety purposes, liver enzyme tests
should be run prior to initiation of treatment and monthly throughout the
course of treatment.

MEDICATION TIPS FOR PATIENTS

In order to get the best results, it is important to take medication exactly as prescribed. Here are some tips that can help you avoid missing doses or forgetting
whether you have taken your medication.

1. Have your health care provider give the medication in a blister card,
labeled so that you will know whether you took each day's dose. If not avail-

able, get a pillbox with compartments for each day, and place the pills into them as soon as your prescription is filled.

2. Take your dose at the same time every day. Make it part of your routine. If you are going to be taking it in the morning and you eat breakfast or have coffee, put the pills on your kitchen table (but out of the reach of young children) and take them with your meal or morning cup of coffee. Or, if you prefer, take them when you brush your teeth in the morning or at night. You can incorporate the medication into any specific routine—such as choosing your clothes in the morning. Just be sure to associate with them with something that you do each and every day.

3. If you feel comfortable about it, ask your partner or spouse to help you remember your medication and to help think of this as part of his or her routine as well.

4. Put a note on your refrigerator, medicine cabinet, or anywhere else that you will see regularly to remind yourself to take your medication. Move the note around so that it does not fade into the background and cease to be an effective reminder.

5. If you feel like deliberately missing a dose, call your health care provider to discuss why. Be honest about feelings related to your illness or your medication (e.g., side effects you are experiencing or concerns about what could happen). Your health care provider can help you work out whether they are related to your medication. Often, just slightly changing the dose can make a difference in your comfort.

6. If the reason you want to skip a dose is because you are experiencing urges to drink or use drugs, call your health care provider or someone you trust from a support group, or an addiction treatment program. The urge will pass—and if you take the medications, it will pass faster.

References

Alcoholics Anonymous. (1976). *The story of how many thousands of men and women have recovered from alcoholism.* New York: Alcoholics Anonymous World Services.

Babor, T.F., J. R. de la Fuente, et al. (1992). *AUDIT: The Alcohol Use Disorders Identification Test: Guidelines for use in primary health care.* Geneva: World Health Organization.

Berg, B. J., H. M. Pettinati, et al. (1996). A risk–benefit assessment of naltrexone in the treatment of alcohol dependence. *Drug Safety* **15**(4): 274–282.

Bien, T. H., W. R. Miller, et al. (1993). Brief interventions for alcohol problems: A review [see comments]. *Addiction* **88**(3): 315–335.

Brown, S. A., A. Gleghorn, et al. (1996). Conduct disorder among adolescent alcohol and drug abusers. *Journal of Studies on Alcohol* **57**(3): 314–324.

Carver, C. S., & R. G. Dunham. (1991). Abstinence expectancy and abstinence among men undergoing inpatient treatment for alcoholism. *Journal of Substance Abuse* **3**(1): 39–57.

Cherpitel, C. J. (1999). Screening for alcohol problems in the U.S. general population: A comparison of the CAGE and TWEAK by gender, ethnicity, and services utilization. *Journal of Studies on Alcohol* **60**(5): 705–711.

Cramer, J. A., R. D. Scheyer, et al. (1990). Compliance declines between clinic visits [see comments]. *Archives of Internal Medicine* **150**(7): 1509–1510.

Crits-Christoph, P., L. Siqueland, et al. (1999). Psychosocial treatments for cocaine dependence: National Institute on Drug Abuse Collaborative Cocaine Treatment Study [see comments]. *Archives of General Psychiatry* **56**(6): 493–502.

Derogatis, L. R., & N. Melisaratps. (1983). The Brief Symptom Inventory: An introductory report. *Psychological Medicine* **13**(3): 595–605.

Gerstein, D. R., & L. S. Lewin. (1990). Treating drug problems. *New England Journal of Medicine* **323**(12): 844–848.

Hayashida, M., A. I. Alterman, et al. (1989). Comparative effectiveness and costs of inpatient and outpatient detoxification of patients with mild-to-moderate alcohol withdrawal syndrome [see comments]. *New England Journal of Medicine* **320**(6): 358–365.

Hester, R. K., & W. R. Miller. (1995). *Handbook of alcoholism treatment approaches: Effective alternatives.* Boston: Allyn & Bacon.

Irvin, J. E., C. A. Bowers, et al. (1999). Efficacy of relapse prevention: A meta-analytic review. *Journal of Consulting and Clinical Psychology* **67**(4): 563–570.

Kaempf, G., C. O'Donnell, et al. (1999). The BRENDA model: A psychosocial addiction model to identify and treat alcohol disorders in elders. *Geriatric Nursing* **20**: 302–304.

Kranzler, H. R., J. A. Burleson, et al. (1994). Buspirone treatment of anxious alcoholics: A placebo-controlled trial. *Archives of General Psychiatry* **51**(9): 720–731.

Larimer, M. E., & G. A. Marlatt. (1990). Applications of relapse prevention with moderation goals. *Journal of Psychoactive Drugs* **22**(2): 189–195.

Mayfield, D., G. McLeod, et al. (1974). The CAGE questionnaire: Validation of a new alcoholism screening instrument. *American Journal of Psychiatry* **131**(10): 1121–1123.

McLellan, A. T., I. O. Arndt, et al. (1993). The effects of psychosocial services in substance abuse treatment [see comments]. *Journal of the American Medical Association* **269**(15): 1953–1959.

Michael, J., & S. Jones. (1999). *The art of moderation: An alternative to alcoholism.* San Francisco: Vision Books International.

Miller, W. R. (1995). Increasing motivation to change. In *Handbook of alcoholism treatment: Effective alternatives* (R. K. Hester & W. R. Miller, Eds.). Boston: Allyn & Bacon: 89–104.

Miller, W. R. (1998). Why do people change addictive behavior?: The 1996 H. David Archibald Lecture. *Addiction* **93**(2): 163–172.

Miller, W. R., R. G. Benefield, et al. (1993). Enhancing motivation for change in problem drinking: A controlled comparison of two therapist styles. *Journal of Consulting and Clinical Psychology* **61**(3): 455–461.

Morse, R. M., & D. K. Flavin. (1992). The definition of alcoholism. The Joint Committee of the National Council on Alcoholism and Drug Dependence and the American Society of Addiction Medicine to study the definition and criteria for the diagnosis of alcoholism [see comments]. *Journal of the American Medical Association* **268**: 1012–1014.

O'Brien, C. P. (1997). Progress in the science of addiction [editorial comment] [see comments]. *American Journal of Psychiatry* **154**(9): 1195–1197.

O'Malley, S. S. (1995). Integration of opioid antagonists and psychosocial therapy in the treatment of alcohol dependence. *Journal of Clinical Psychiatry* **56**(Suppl., 7): 30–38.

Pettinati, H. M., J. R. Volpicelli, et al. (2000). Improving naltrexone response: An intervention for medical practitioners to enhance medication in alcohol dependent patients. *Journal of Addictive Diseases* **19**: 71–83.

Prochaska, J. O., & C. C. DiClemente. (1983). Stages and processes of self-change of smoking: Toward an integrative model of change. *Journal of Consulting and Clinical Psychology* **51**(3): 390–395.

Prochaska, J. O., C. C. DiClemente, et al. (1992). In search of how people change: Applications to addictive behaviors. *American Psychologist* **47**(9): 1102–1114.

Prochaska, J. O., J. C. Norcross, et al. (1994). *Changing for good.* New York: HarperCollins.

Project MATCH Research Group. (1997). Matching alcoholism treatments to client heterogeneity: Project MATCH posttreatment drinking outcomes [see comments]. *Journal of Studies on Alcohol* **58**(1): 7–29.

Salzman, C. (1995). Medication compliance in the elderly. *Journal of Clinical Psychiatry* **56**: 18–22.

Schuckit, M. A., J. Klein, et al. (1994). Personality test scores as predictors of alcoholism almost a decade later. *American Journal of Psychiatry* **151**(7): 1038–1042.

Schuckit, M. A., J. E. Tipp, & T. L. Smith. (1997). Periods of abstinence following the onset of alcohol dependence in 1,853 men and women. *Journal of Studies on Alcohol* **58**(6): 581–589.

Vaillant, G. E. (1996). A long-term follow-up of male alcohol abuse. *Archives of General Psychiatry* **53**(3): 243–249.

Volpicelli, J. R., K. C. Rhines, et al. (1997). Naltrexone and alcohol dependence: Role of subject compliance [see comments]. *Archives of General Psychiatry* **54**(8): 737–742.

Volpicelli, J., & M. Szalavitz. (2000). *Recovery options: The complete guide.* New York: Wiley.

Woody, G. E., A. T. McLellan, et al. (1990). Psychotherapy and counseling for methadone-maintained opiate addicts: Results of research studies. *NIDA Research Monographs* **104**: 9–23.

Index

Alcoholics Anonymous, assumptions
    (*continued*)
    alcoholics need improved spiri-
        tual/moral condition for self-
        esteem, 7–8
    alcoholism is a chronic disease, 8,
        73
    characteristics of successful
        patients, 72
    comparison with BRENDA model,
        10, 11*t*
    cause of substance abuse, 10–11
    desired outcome, 14
    level of care, 11–12
    practitioners, 13
    psychosocial support, 15
    research support, 14–15
    treatment and its duration, 12
    use of medications, 12–13, 78
    view of relapse, 13–14
    HALT common triggers, 107–108,
        107t, 153
    inpatient facilities, 73
    rank as treatment option, 74
    relapse prevention techniques, 73
    variations, 76
Anhedonia
    and antidepressants, 97
    and naltrexone, 95–96
    as a relapse trigger, 103

Biopsychosocial assessment, *see also*
    BRENDA model/stages
    approach
    special issues in initial presenta-
        tion for treatment, 35–39
    importance of nonjudgmental atti-
        tude, 36, 39
    conducting the comprehensive
        evaluation, 39
    collaboration between health care
        professionals, 42–43
    key areas, 40*t*–42*t*
        biological assessment, 40*t*, 43–44
        psychological assessment, 41*t*,
            44–45
        social assessment, 41*t*–42*t*, 46
    dimensions to measure severity of
        problems, 49
    screening for addiction, 33–35

Biopsychosocial model of addictions,
    3, *see also* BRENDA
    elements incorporated from
        traditional models, 9
Blood screens for drugs/alcohol, and
    patient's permission, 44
BRENDA model, 10, 31*t*, *see also*
    Alcoholics Anonymous/Minnesota
    Model/Comparison with BRENDA
    addressing denial of disorder, 24
    as brief intervention to initiate
        treatment, 26
    comparison with other models, 78
    components, and criteria for
        component completion, 121–123
    course of treatment, 127, *see also*
        Typical course of treatment/
        BRENDA model
    and establishment of collaborative
        therapeutic alliance, 17, 24–25
    implementation prerequisites, 30
    and integration with Stages of
        Change model, 21–23
    as a patient centered approach, 16,
        62, 118
    and phamacotherapy integration
        education on specific medication,
            92
        monitoring pill counts, 92
        proactively addressing patient is-
            sues of medication adherence,
            92–93
    stages, 4, 17, 20–21, *see also*
        Recovery, early recovery phase
        issues/BRENDA model
    Biopsychosocial evaluation stage,
        17–18, *see also*
        Biopsychosocial assessment
    Report to patient, 18, 24, *see also*
        Report of Assessment Results
    Empathetic understanding, 18, *see
        also* Empathic listening
    Needs expressed by patient, 18–
        19, 22, 25, *see also* Needs/pri-
        orities (patient's) identification
    Direct advice, 19, 24–25, *see also*
        Direct advice/guidance
    Assess patient's responses, 19–20,
        see also Patient's response as-
        sessment

Prochaska, James, *see* Motivational interviewing
Psychological Symptom Inventory–32, 45

Rational Recovery, *see* Addiction treatments/mutual self-help groups
Recovery
early recovery phase issues, 101, 103*t*
and BRENDA model, 102
importance of employment, 112
protracted withdrawal symptoms, 103
later recovery phase issues, 114–115, 115*t*
and BRENDA model, 122–123
childhood issues, 117
less intensive role for practitioner, 122
life changes, 117–118
triggers reexamination, 115–116
"recovery jobs, " 112
Relapse, 23
in early recovery phase, 102
vs. lapse, 108
in Moderation Management, 108–112
process, 103–104
triggers, 103, *see also* Recovery/ later phase issues
HALT (hungry, angry, lonely, tired), 107, 107–108
identifying underlying needs, 104–105
learning protective techniques, 105–107
(sexual) partner issues, 112–113
in later recovery phase, 119–121
awareness of indicators, 119–121
case example, 173
"cure" misconception, 119, 121
as a process, 119
Report of Assessment Results, 47–48, *see also* BRENDA model/stages
applying empathy, 57
challenging fear-eliciting assumptions, 58–59
collaboration, 60–61
coping with anxiety, 57–58

fear ambivalence to preparation, 59–60
assess reaction to report/stage of change, 51–54
profile formulation
drug/alcohol addiction question, 48–49
severity of biopsychosocial complications, 49–50
dimensions of severity, 49
results reporting, 50–51
"Rock bottom" concept, and BRENDA model, 66

Sanchez-Craig, Martha, *see* Drink-Wise Program
Secular Organizations for Sobriety, *see* Addiction treatments/mutual self-help groups
Sexual activity issues, in early recovery, 112–113
SMART Recovery, *see* Addiction treatments/mutual self-help groups
Substance Use Disorders Screen, 187–189

Temperance Movement, 6–7
Treatment, *see also* Addiction treatment; Typical course of treatment/BRENDA model
Treatment compliance, 23–25
Trimpey, Jack, and Rational Recovery, 77
12-step programs, 72–74, *see also* Alcoholics Anonymous/Minnesota model
Typical course of treatment/BRENDA model
cocaine and alcohol addiction with severe complications, 127, 161–162
initiating treatment
focus on addiction screening/biopsychosocial evaluation/patient safety needs, 144–146
focus on direct advice, 146–148
focus on empathetic understanding, 148–150
early recovery phase
BRENDA evaluations, 150–156